Contents

The sociology of mental disorder

**International Library of Sociology
and Social Reconstruction**

Founded by Karl Mannheim
Editor: W. J. H. Sprott

A catalogue of the books available in the **International Library of Sociology
and Social Reconstruction,** and new books in preparation for the Library will
be found at the end of this volume.

The sociology of mental disorder

Roger Bastide

translated by Jean McNeil

London   Routledge & Kegan Paul

First published in Great Britain 1972
by Routledge & Kegan Paul Ltd.
Broadway House, 68–74 Carter Lane,
London EC4V 5EL
Printed in Great Britain by Western Printing Services Ltd, Bristol

Original French Edition *Sociologie des Maladies Mentales*
© Flammarion, Paris, 1965
Translated from the French by Jean McNeil
© Routledge & Kegan Paul, 1972
No part of this book may be repoduced in
any form without the permission from the
publisher, except for the quotation of
brief passages in criticism

ISBN 0 7100 6974 x

List of diagrams

List of tables

Introduction

In the past few years a completely new field of research has emerged which has generally been called 'social psychiatry'. Nothing could obviously be more exciting than to explore unknown territory and to blaze trails through the ill-defined borderland between two sciences, psychiatry and sociology. Even a mistake can lead to success, and getting lost only means discovering new lands. At some point, however, disorganized research ceases to be productive and actually becomes detrimental: we find each person concentrating on the bit of territory he has claimed and maintaining that it is the only one that can be called 'social psychiatry'; the territories partly overlap, and the jungle gives way to a chaotic patchwork of cultivated fields with ill-defined boundaries impinging on each other. It is time to draw up a land register, which is no easy task.

We need only open a book on social psychiatry to be aware of the haziness of the definitions used. If we try to be more precise we end up with almost as many definitions as there are authors; worse still, some authors give different names to the same field of research, as though two explorers in our jungle had inadvertently taken over the same land and each named it after his own ruler. A whole book could be written on social psychiatry on the same lines as Kroeber's and Kluckhohn's work on the concepts and definitions of the term 'culture' if we were to collect these different meanings and try to classify them in broad categories according to the authors' nationality or orientation.[1] It will be sufficient, however, to mention the principal definitions in use.

The first definition gives social psychiatry the essential aim of studying the methods by which society combats mental disorder. Psychosis and neurosis are treated as 'social problems', along with crime, unemployment and divorce.[2] The present increase in the number of mental patients can be interpreted in two different

1

ways: either as a real increase, due to economic crises and world wars, or as an apparent one, due simply to changing social structures and values which mean that patients are no longer cared for at home, but in institutions. In either case this increase raises serious problems for governments. Which methods of therapy and prevention should be applied? Should patients be isolated or rehabilitated? What is the cost of these various measures? In this sense social psychiatry is a branch of social pathology—as defined by the Americans—and of applied sociology. Workers in this field are becoming more and more numerous, due to increasing interest in the under-developed countries and in 'world health'; they are particularly concerned with the difficulties encountered in the application of mental-health policies and the evaluation of different solutions.

A second and equally pragmatic definition akin to but different from the first is the one given by such authors as Adler[3] and Hartwell:[4] social psychiatry is the psychiatric training given to social workers. It is obvious that the psychiatric hospital is unlike other hospitals, where the patient, though bedridden, is still part of society. The psychiatric hospital is a 'community' where the patient learns to readjust to life in society and to regain his feeling of moral responsibility and his sense of independence. Therefore, in this case the nurses and social workers perform particular functions which require specialized training. The term 'social psychiatry'—that is, psychiatric treatment aimed at the patient's reintegration into society—may be the best possible term to use in this context.

There is a third definition which is close to the second and even partly overlaps it: Maxwell Jones[5] has used the term 'social psychiatry' in connection with the therapeutic community, the re-establishment of social relationships, the socialization of the isolate and, in particular, with group therapy and occupational therapy. Here the function of social psychiatry is to evaluate the various methods of social rehabilitation, such as Moreno's psychodrama, group dynamics, recreational and work groups, etc.

As defined so far, social psychiatry appears to be more of a practical science than a theoretical one. It is understandable that such definitions should tend to be the work of psychiatrists rather than sociologists: they reflect the growing feeling that society, although it may have to protect itself against all disruptive factors, also has a duty towards the mentally ill, and that we cannot leave it to chance or to trial-and-error methods to discover the remedies. A pragmatic approach is increasingly giving way to a planned approach, and it would seem that social psychiatry as defined above corresponds to this need for planned mental-health policies.

But any art or practical science must be preceded by a theoretical science. This theoretical science will be all the more productive if the scientist is able to detach himself as much as possible from its potential applications, so as to avoid being disturbed by the feelings, ideas and values of his social group and to make objectivity his sole aim. The sociology of knowledge has made us familiar with the idea that even the 'objective' scientist is influenced by his class and racial prejudices. Le Guillant wondered whether the refusal of French psychiatrists to accept social psychiatry was not due to a *bourgeois* reluctance to admit that society could play a part in the causation of mental illness. In choosing to consider only the neurological or biological causes of insanity, are we in fact shunning our responsibilities as members of society? Whatever our feelings may be on this point, which we cannot develop here, we now come to a set of definitions of social psychiatry which are no longer practical, but theoretical. Let us examine them briefly.

First of all, for a number of research workers social psychiatry is the study of the role of social factors in the causation of mental disorder. We owe to social psychology the knowledge that man cannot exist outside society, that the personality is shaped by and within social groups, that the concept of ego and the concept of alter ego develop side by side, and that individual and social factors are closely interwoven. Social psychiatry is simply the extension of this principle from normal to pathological man. It is possible, of course, as did Henri Ey in France, to recognize social psychology and not social psychiatry. What is more, the recognition of social influences need not mean the ruling out of such physiological factors as heredity, innate predisposition, brain damage, etc. Nor does it mean that the therapist should neglect the physical and chemical treatment of mental illness in favour of psychotherapy or sociotherapy. Social psychiatry in the present sense is the study of social influences (family structure, housing conditions, economic status, occupational stress, religion, etc.) in the causation of behaviour disorders. This is the most generally accepted definition. Marvin K. Opler, for example, defines social psychiatry as the study of the aetiology and dynamics of mental disorder seen in their social and cultural environment. He points out that human behaviour cannot be understood in isolation from the environment, which impinges on the psyche and therefore on the soma. Pavlov demonstrated this in showing the role of learning and conditioned responses. But it is important to add here that man does not merely respond to external stimuli: he also interprets them. Unlike animals, he reacts not only to signals but to symbols.[6]

Precisely because this is the most generally accepted definition of social psychiatry, it is also perhaps the most confused and

3

tangled one. Some authors, such as Sullivan,[7] think that the individual cannot be considered outside the framework of his personal relations, and that the psychiatrist must therefore seek the help of the sociologist. Others, such as Masserman,[8] think that psychiatrists should incorporate sociology in a dynamic study of the morbid personality. The social factor is not outside the subject, an influence acting on him from without; it is experienced in a particular way by each individual and can only be apprehended from the inside, by the psyche. Yet others, such as Opler,[9] warn of the dangers of separating social from cultural influences, and of the psychiatrist concerning himself exclusively with social structure and interaction systems without taking into account the cultural dimension of human behaviour: psychosis and neurosis vary both in incidence and in epidemiology, according to the civilization; abnormal manifestations, like normal ones, have their own patterns and norms. Later we shall attempt to put some order into these various approaches. For the time being let us note that the present definition of social psychiatry embraces work as different as that of Faris and Dunham on the distribution of mental illness according to ecological area in Chicago,[10] which is sociology, the work of Devereux on psychiatric disturbance among the Mohave Indians,[11] which is anthropology, and that of Dollard and his collaborators on the relation between aggression and social frustration,[12] which is social psychology. We could also add such studies as Valabrega's on the therapeutic relationship, which are psychological studies of interaction or interpersonal relations between the psychiatrist and the patient.[13]

In short, it is possible to distinguish two interwoven meanings within this one definition, one for psychiatrists and the other for sociologists. The psychiatrist is interested only in the individual, and therefore his method is the clinical or case-study method; he is concerned with weighing up the respective influence of various social factors in causing the disturbance of a particular patient. At the extreme limit, social psychiatry amounts to what Ombredane calls 'medical psychology' or even to what used to be known in the days of Ribot, Dumas and many others as 'psychopathology'. The sociologist, on the other hand, is only interested in groups. His preferred method is the statistical one, and his aim is to establish correlations between the incidence of mental disorder in a given society and particular elements of this society: ecological areas, class structure, family structure, religious affiliation, etc., treated as so many variables.

Besides this first theoretical meaning we sometimes find another definition which is less frequently used: social psychiatry is the study of pathological communities. But here we are also faced with viewpoints which vary greatly, depending on the author. Some believe there is such a thing as mass neurosis, and they like to quote the example of Nazism in Germany; in this case social psychiatry means the study of sickness in social groups and psychiatry proper is the study of sickness in the individual. Many psychiatrists, however, do not accept the idea of collective neurosis and still less of collective psychosis. They maintain that only individuals can actually be ill, but they do believe in the possibility of mental contagion and the occurrence of epidemics, such as the famous epidemics of mystical insanity in the Middle Ages. Social psychiatry would, therefore, study the laws or the mechanics of contamination and propagation, the ways in which mental illness is transmitted from the individual to the collectivity, and the social factors which favour this transmission. It is thus possible to differentiate between the psychiatry of the individual, the psychiatry of two people in interaction (*folie à deux*) and the psychiatry of more than two people (*folie multiple*).

Quite apart from collective neurosis, one can also include in social psychiatry, as Baruk has done, the study of processes regarded as pathological which can affect the way in which society reacts to the individual, and processes of change which are considered morbid, e.g. the transition from community to society (in so far as it implies a transition from moral pressures to social sanctions), or the development of such phenomena as the power cult, inhuman bureaucratization, arbitrary arrests, increasing contempt for the sick and the old and worship of the State. Social psychiatry is then identified with the study of the 'sickness of society'; however, it is different from 'social pathology' in that it is interested in the individual and the ways in which he is afflicted and demoralized by these sicknesses.[14]

Still in the theoretical field, we find one last and even rarer meaning of the term. It is the theoretical counterpart of social psychiatry in the sense of group therapy: the study of the social behaviour of the mentally ill. The study of small groups has become an important part of American sociology; it is also possible to form small experimental groups with mental patients—either homogeneous groups, composed, for example, of paranoid patients, or heterogeneous groups. Within these groups particular phenomena can be studied, such as the emergence of leaders, the resolution of tension, the formation of group consciousness. It is then possible to manipulate a variety of factors, from external ones, such as the social-class composition of the group, to internal ones, such as the respective position of the patients within the group (around the table, in relation to the psychiatrist, etc.).

It is clear that from the moment social psychiatry was recognized as a new scientific field it was explored in many different ways, according to the interests of the investigators or their desire to break new ground, leaving us in the end with an ill-assorted mess of definitions. This process could hardly have taken place without some conflict. The conflicts are interesting since they show an awareness of the necessity to untangle the muddle and put some order into a confusion of heterogeneous and even contradictory definitions. Thus Deshaies in France considers that the study of collective psychosis or neurosis is not social psychiatry, but social pathology; the term 'social psychiatry' should only be applied to the study of the social aspect of mental illness.[15] Eliot suggests that the term 'socio-analysis' or 'psychiatric sociology' (not to be confused with social psychiatry, to which he gives an altogether different meaning) should be applied to mental-hygiene practices, psychiatric social work or psychiatric social work training.[16] These conflicts are a sign that we have reached a point in the history of social psychiatry where it is necessary to draw up what we earlier described as a land register of the occupied territory.

But most research workers would not like to lose any of this wealth of definitions, and they feel that the best way to put some order into the situation is to make each of the approaches we have briefly mentioned so far into a special branch of a comprehensive discipline. Thus Baruk places social psychiatry at the meeting-point of two aspects of psychopathology: it studies both the social causes of insanity and the social consequences of individual neuroses and psychoses. It includes individual psychopathology (guilt feelings, the over-developed conscience of the melancholic, disturbances of volition, etc.) as well as the psychopathology of society.[17] Hans Strozka defines the field of social psychiatry as (1) the study of the rehabilitation of mental patients through work, family care and hospital treatment, (2) the study of the influence of social factors in the aetiology of mental disorder, (3) the study of group therapy, and (4) the study of the cultural dimension in the epidemiology of mental disorder. The intention is clearly to allow for the co-existence, by calling them separate branches, of the various fields where research has already been done. Strozka quotes the work of Rennie, Bierer, Maxwell and Erikson, among others, without worrying about whether they belong to the same discipline or to different disciplines which would then have to be split into various fields.[18] Schermerhorn is, in our opinion, much more systematic: he tries to give the different fields he encounters a logical order, so that social psychiatry should still retain a certain unity. He thinks that the term 'social psychiatry' should first of all be applied to the study of the social and cultural dimensions of mental disorder. Thus the lower classes are said to exhibit relatively more conduct disorders, the middle classes more psychosomatic disorders associated with repression or social control, and the upper classes more psychoneuroses and manic-depressive psychoses. Next it is to be applied to the study of therapy as a social relationship: this would consist in examining, under a different heading for each aspect that has been explored, (1) the therapeutic relationship between doctor and patient, (2) group therapy regarded as an experimental study of small groups rather than in its practical aspect, and (3) the mental hospital as a social institution characterized by the disappearance of sexual and family relationships and of the occupational life of the mental patient, who enters into a new system of interrelations with nurses, doctors, the hospital administration and a heterogeneous mass of mental patients. The last function of social psychiatry, its practical application, in fact, is the study of the prevention of mental illness and the planning of mental-health policies for various types of community (urban, rural or under-developed).[19]

These attempts to unite within the same field such apparently unrelated phenomena as the distribution of mental illness according to social class and the organization of a mental hospital are not without interest. However, we believe that, given the present state of research, the best approach is to pulverize the concept of social psychiatry, to break it down, rather than to stretch it indefinitely to cover so many different phenomena.

To begin with, if we look at the history of social psychiatry, we find that it was developed by different scientists in different countries, who were unaware of each other's existence, and who gave the term very different meanings. To try to find an *a posteriori* common denominator is more of a game than a serious enterprise. Secondly, it is important to note that the word 'social' is ambiguous, and covers a whole range of meanings from those containing a value judgment to those which stem from the birth of scientific sociology. Does 'social' in the term 'social psychiatry' mean 'appertaining to society' or 'of a sociological character or nature'? Finally and most important, the various approaches of social psychiatrists can only be brought together through the common ground of psychiatry. The common factor in most of the research we have mentioned so far is that it has been done by psychiatrists either working alone or in a team with other social scientists.

But the expression 'social psychiatry' is composed of two terms, 'social' and 'psychiatry'. If we consider the first term, we necessarily think of the various disciplines which from different points of view are concerned with mental illness: social psychology, sociology, anthropology. Why give the second term more importance than the first? Surely it is the first term which gives meaning to the second, which makes it specific. Since the first is more important than the second, would it not be better to distinguish three fields—social psychology, the sociology of mental disorder and the anthropology of mental disorder—since present-day students are unlikely to confuse social psychology, sociology and anthropology, in spite of the fact that all three are interrelated.

It seems that much confusion and many spurious problems would be avoided, as well as conflicts between research workers (American sociologists often complain of the authoritarian attitude of psychiatrists as collaborators), if one were carefully to delineate and separate the various fields, giving them each a different name. In any case, we are not dealing with a simple question of terminology. Behind the terminology there is a set of distinct and independent sciences of man or of society, with their own methods, their own ways of approaching facts and their own theoretical conceptualizations.

We would be in favour of reserving the term 'social psychiatry' for the study of the morbid social behaviour of mentally disturbed persons. This is in a sense what Krout suggested as early as 1933 when he gave social psychiatry the aim of discovering and controlling the social causes of mental disorder.[20] The accent is then placed on psychopathology rather than on sociology. If this definition is accepted, social psychology becomes a particular branch of social psychology. Social psychology proper is therefore the study of the normal personality and social psychiatry is that of the abnormal personality; the first is concerned with the individual's socialization and the second with his desocialization. It is for this very reason that American social psychiatry textbooks always include at least one chapter on 'the pathological forms of consciousness' (Bernard)[21] or 'social psychopathology' (Klineberg),[22] which summarizes the principal conclusions of social psychiatry.

The sociology of mental disorder would then be an entirely separate field, solely concerned with communities and groups. When Auguste Comte accused doctors of being mere veterinarians of the human body, whereas man is both a biological and a social being, he laid the foundations of social psychiatry. On the other hand, when his disciple, Audiffrend, pointed out that the disorganization of the personality accompanies the disorganization of society, that a distinction can be made between organic periods where mental disorder is at a minimum, and periods of crisis where it is at a maximum, he laid the foundations of the sociology of mental disorder. To give only a few examples: Krout's social psychiatry comes close to social psychology while the social psychiatry of Dunham, Brown or Felson is definitely well within the field of sociology. Let us note in passing that this distinction removes at least one possibility of confusion. The social psychiatrist is often faced with the question of the existence of reactive psychosis. The part played by social factors and social causes has to be assessed. But the sociologist can avoid the problem of aetiology. He can establish correlations between certain social phenomena and certain types of illness without stating whether they necessarily represent causal relationships. The sociology of mental disorder, as distinct from social psychiatry, can therefore benefit more easily from the wealth of material available today on methodology and systematization in the field of sociology.

Earlier we linked the concept of social psychiatry in its narrowest sense with that of psychopathology. Should we now do the same for what we have termed the sociology of mental disorder and social pathology? It is obvious that when such psychiatrists as Baruk or Veil—to choose two widely different scientists—study phenomena of social pathology they employ a different approach than that of the sociologist, and can provide him with new insights. In our opinion, however, the sociology of mental disorder can only constitute one branch of social pathology, along with many other fields, such as criminology, the study of the disorganization of the family, anomie, etc. But, on the other hand, social pathology cannot be reduced to the equivalent of social psychiatry or to a mere branch of social psychiatry. We would like to suggest that the sociology of mental disorder be considered rather as a particular branch of sociology. It would be more appropriate to compare it to what is known as medical sociology, which examines similar problems in relation to such illnesses as venereal disease, tuberculosis, epidemics and to general problems of health.

We would equally include in the sociology of mental disorder two other spheres of study which are also essentially sociological, but which are related to other branches of traditional sociology. First of all, group therapy in so far as its theoretical aspect is given more importance than its practical aspect; it would therefore be linked to what the Americans call the 'sociology of small groups'. Secondly, the study of the organization of mental hospitals, of the interaction between administration, doctors, nursing staff and patients. The mental hospital does have distinctive features, and its patients are different from other patients; nevertheless, it can be included in the study of the hospital as an institution, a field of increasing interest to sociologists. This field can be regarded as part of the sociology of institutions, initiated by the school of Le Play, with its monographs on industrial firms.

Finally, we come to the anthropology of mental disorder, which we will call 'ethnopsychiatry' (not as a branch of ethnopsychology, either normal or pathological, but of anthropology). It is necessary here to make a number of distinctions. The study of the cultural dimension as a factor in individual mental disturbance is pathological ethnopsychology, and consequently, according to our preceding definitions, belongs to the field of social psychiatry. But if our aim is to establish correlations between particular ethnic factors (such as the composition or structure of the family, stratification systems, the importance or the function of religion and magic in a society, age grades, etc.) and types of mental illness, or the symptoms that characterize them, then our field of study is that of traditional anthropology. But there is another aspect of ethnopsychiatry of even more interest to the anthropologist, or, if one prefers, even more distinctly anthropological, which consists in compiling what Devereux called 'psychiatry textbooks' for the primitive societies studied. That is to say, not to rethink native concepts, using the concepts of Western psychiatry, or to establish the correlations mentioned above, but to look at the original classifications of mental disturbance made by the natives, their distinctive aetiology and the way in which these disturbances are treated and cured.[23]

To each of these three theoretical disciplines there naturally corresponds a practical application. We can accept Thomas D. Eliot's term, although it is not, in my opinion, ideal, 'psychiatric sociology', on condition that we add the adjective 'applied'.[24] It would encompass all fields from group therapy to community health projects onwards. One of its aspects would relate to social psychiatry (group therapy, readjustment of discharged mental patients to work and social life, reorganization of the hospital system), one to the sociology of mental disorder (preventive measures, town planning, mental hygiene, and also the reorganization of the hospital system), and the third to anthropology (mental-health projects in underdeveloped countries or rural communities).

In short, we suggest a threefold division, each science to have its practical extensions, rather than a single field. This is because in the term 'social psychiatry' the word 'social' seems more important than the word 'psychiatry', and also because the qualities required of the research worker, his method of approach and his conceptualizations are different in each of the three fields: social psychiatry proper (or social psychopathology), the sociology of mental disorder and ethnopsychiatry. One more question remains unanswered: Why, in spite of all this, is there such a blind attachment to the concept of a single field? Historical contingencies and the fact that psychiatrists are present in all three disciplines, in collaboration with social psychologists, sociologists and anthropologists, still do not account for this situation. So now that we have made this threefold division we must try to see what are the avenues of communication between our three distinct fields. A land register does not prevent neighbours from entertaining co-operative relations; on the contrary, it makes it easier and we have personally struggled long enough for the promotion of interdisciplinary research to welcome the setting up of these avenues of communication.

Whether social psychiatry applies the ideas of sociology, as Sullivan did, or whether it encompasses them, as the school of dynamic psychiatry does, it remains true that social psychiatry presupposes the establishment of a sociology of mental disorder. On the other hand, anthropology enables the psychiatrist to see the importance of the cultural dimension in the morbid personality. It reveals to him that mental disturbance is as inextricably linked to the world of values (or, according to Karen Horney, to the conflict of values) as it is to the world of symbols. Similarly, the sociologist studying mental illness cannot do without the help of social psychiatry, the statistical method only giving fruitful results if it is completed by the case history. Statistics may show, for example, that schizophrenics tend to be concentrated in districts containing hotels and guest-houses, but they cannot tell us whether the schizophrenic's handicap leads him to seek a place where he can live in isolation or whether, on the contrary, it is the environmental setting which has an effect on the disorganization of his personality. The same can be said of ethnopsychiatry. The psychiatrist who chooses to work outside Western society needs to become familiar with the customs, norms and social structure of the country he is living in; for example, transference in the therapeutic relationship will take on different forms according to whether the authority figure is the father or the maternal uncle. Paranoid tendencies can be masked in primitive societies by magical rites and can consequently be difficult to detect by contrasting them with normal institutionalized behaviour. The sick person is not alienated as in our society, but is integrated with the group, although he remains sick. In return, the anthropologist needs to be familiar with research in social psychiatry. Note, for example, the important part played by social psychiatry in the formation of the particular school which focused its attention on the relation between 'culture and personality'. The distinction between 'shame cultures' and 'guilt cultures', based on the exteriorization or internalization of social control, is as fundamental to the anthropologist as it is to the psychiatrist. Co-operation is obviously essential between the three disciplines.

The present work only intends to tackle one of these three disciplines: the sociology of mental disorder. But because of the interrelations between this particular field as we have defined it and social psychiatry and ethnopsychiatry, it will be necessary to indicate the avenues which lead imperceptibly from one field to another.

For example, to move from correlation to causal explanation means to go from sociology to social psychiatry, or to emphasize the cultural dimension in psychic disorders means applying to Western society the postulates of ethnopsychiatry. We shall confine ourselves as far as possible to indicating these avenues of communication rather than following them up.

The book is divided into three main parts. We shall first of all tackle the more general questions relating to the theory and method of the sociology of mental disorder. We will then give an account of the different empirical studies which have been made in this field. Finally, we shall outline a 'structural' thesis to give a better theoretical framework to a discipline which is today in rapid growth.

I The formation and development of a sociology of mental disorder

1 The foundations of the sociology of mental disorder

The sociology of mental disorder is often thought to be a new science. In reality it is as old as sociology itself, since Comte was the founder of both.

Comte was as critical of doctors as he was of lawyers: 'they only study the animal in us'. In other words, they deserve the title of 'veterinarian', rather than of 'doctor'. He was the forerunner of psychosomatic medicine in two senses. First, in the emphasis he placed on the interaction of mental and physical phenomena: 'As man is the most indivisible of beings, unless his body and soul are studied simultaneously, the ideas we form about him can only be mistaken or superficial.' Second, in his linking of medicine with the priesthood and consequently with the 'Religion of Humanity'.[1] It is surprising to find the word 'soul' used by an opponent of psychology—a science which he divided into two fields, one belonging to biology and the other to sociology. The doctor who only sees in man a body is a veterinarian; the one who wishes to see both body and soul must necessarily turn to sociology. What, then, are the contributions of sociology to the study of mental illness?

We find scattered elements of a sociology of mental disorder in Comte's writing, but it was his disciple, Audiffrend, who, by attempting to systematize Comte's theories, first produced a coherent positivist picture of mental disorder. Roughly speaking, he says that insanity is characterized by a twofold 'subjectivity', both logical and social. From the point of view of logic, insanity, like the dream and the day-dream, is a process without object, whereas the scientific or positive approach is dependent on the object. From the social viewpoint, insanity, again like the dream and the day-dream, represents the mind which has broken away

13

from collective control, which is given over to itself, to the amorality of its inner world and the unleashing of its desires. In Comte's words, insanity is the mind in a state of 'selfishness', the revolt of the individual against humanity. The revolt against objective reality and the revolt against altruism are not basically different, but represent the same process, the surrender of the individual to 'subjectivity'.

This surrender characterizes certain periods in history: insanity has always existed, but its incidence varies according to the period. Thus we find in Comte's work not only a sociological definition of insanity, but also a study of the sociological conditions associated with its appearance. Positivism distinguishes between organic periods and periods of crisis, according to whether solidarity between individuals is organized or whether it is in the process of disintegrating. For instance, the Middle Ages are an organic period, and the age of Positivism is another. But between organic periods there must necessarily be transition periods when one social structure has disintegrated because it no longer corresponds to man's needs and a new structure has not yet emerged. In crisis periods, such as the Reformation or the French Revolution, the individual rebels with the aim of asserting his personal identity. This is when subjectivity, which until then was under the control both of reality and society, makes its appearance. The increase in the incidence of insanity is related to the passing from an organic period into a crisis period and develops alongside, and for the same reasons, as 'individualism'.[2]

It is obvious that Comte's theory, as adopted and transposed into the psychiatric field by Audiffrend, has relevant aspects; it will appear several times in this historical summary—for example, with reference to the work of Charles Blondel. However, it is marred by the confusion Comte makes between subjectivity and individualism. The latter concept, far from being characteristic of a lack of solidarity, indicates on the contrary a different type of solidarity. Since the work of Tönnies in Germany and Durkheim in France, evidence of this fact has been given. The solidarity which Durkheim calls 'organic' as opposed to 'mechanical', and which is founded on the recognition of the rights of the individual, is obviously the more precarious of the two. However, the causes of insanity can be said to lie, not in individualism, which necessarily brings about solidarity, but in the lack of organization of this new type of solidarity. From Durkheim onwards the problem of the sociological origins of insanity is formulated in terms of a new concept, social anomie, to which we shall return shortly.

Morel, author of the *Traité des dégénérescences de l'espèce humaine*, stands in opposition to Comte and Audiffrend. He relates the rise in crime, a phenomenon of social pathology, to the rise in mental disorder, a phenomenon of mental pathology. He does not reach the conclusion that all criminals are mentally abnormal, but he is convinced that there is a connection between these two facts. Man's nervous system is the weakest part of his organism, and can easily be intoxicated by malaria, lead-poisoning, alcohol, etc., thus producing insanity. Society is composed of individuals, the intoxication of whose nervous systems can lead to feeble-mindedness, sterility or criminality. In other words, the degeneration of the individual leads to the degeneration of the race, and eventually to the end of civilization itself. People known as 'primitive' are merely people whose progress has been halted or who have regressed owing to their unhealthy environment and the illnesses caused by it. Morel is in direct opposition to Comte: whereas Comte demonstrated the influence of social factors on mental illness, thereby founding what is known today as the socio-genetic theory, Morel was concerned to show the effects of mental illness, or of any sort of illness on society; he thus established a biogenetic theory of social pathology. But Morel wrote before the appearance of Darwin's work. He based his theory of degeneration on the dogma of the immutability of the species, believing that there existed a normal type of man, but that this type could be affected by disease and corrupted. The disintegration of the nervous system was thus the cause of the disintegration of social ties.

After Darwin the degeneration theory could only survive with some changes. The concept of degeneration was replaced by that of regression. The disintegration of mental functions follows the opposite direction to evolution—that is, the most highly evolved levels are the first to be impaired and the most automatic the last (cf. Jackson in psychiatry, Ribot in psychopathology). Richard drew sociological conclusions from this theory in a series of unpublished lectures. The sicknesses of society are the consequences of regression or disturbances of the will and the personality. The increase in the number of 'amorphous' or 'unstable' people as defined by Ribot is incompatible with a social system which requires increasing determination from the individual.

Thus at its very beginning sociology was already split into two schools, which are still in conflict today: the first looks for social factors in mental disorder and can be traced back to Comte; the second school rejects social factors and tries to define the social effects of the increase in mental illness, and can be traced back to Morel.

2 Crisis in sociology

After Comte French sociology went through a crisis, and it was not until Durkheim and Lévy-Bruhl that it began to come to life again. These two authors marked the transformation of sociology from a more or less philosophical doctrine into a science. What contributions can this science make to our discussion?

Let us start with Lévy-Bruhl. He made a distinction between two types of mentality: the prelogical mentality, characteristic of primitive societies, and the logical mentality, which is that of our society. Could this suggest a promising hypothesis to the psychiatrist? In his study of mental functions in primitive societies, Lévy-Bruhl came up against a difficulty: it was impossible to form an idea of the perception, judgment and actions of primitive man through the intermediary of our own ways of thinking and feeling. The solution he suggested was that strictly objective studies of the primitive mind should take the place of interpretations based on Western thinking. The psychiatrist studying the phenomena of 'morbid consciousness' is faced with the same problem of a way of thinking alien to his own. The solution must therefore be similar: to study morbid consciousness 'as a psychological reality in its own right which is irreducible to our own experience and therefore cannot be reconstructed on the basis of normal states and processes of consciousness'.[3] This was Charles Blondel's approach: he reached the conclusion, contrary, for example, to Ribot, that the difference between the normal and the pathological is not quantitative, but qualitative; morbid consciousness is not a distortion of normal consciousness, but something quite different. Normal consciousness is capable of conceptualization and is therefore socialized, whereas pathological consciousness is incapable of organizing itself according to our 'normal' logical frameworks, of fitting its coenesthetic disturbances into the mould of current language. It is desocialized consciousness.

Thus Blondel and Comte have much in common. Insanity is the triumph of pure subjectivity in its dual departure from reality and from social life. Blondel goes still further, and his ideas lead to a methodological rule: it is impossible to interpret the pathological through the normal. Some critics have accused Blondel of basing his theory on one type of patient only, i.e. those whose disturbances are characterized by anxiety. This criticism does not carry great weight, since Blondel did succeed in throwing light on important phenomena relating to conceptualization and morbid language. In the latter part of this book we shall consider the importance of his contribution. For the time being it will be sufficient to stress the paradoxical quality of a sociological approach whose final result is to challenge the very possibility of a sociology of mental disorder.

Durkheim, as opposed to Lévy-Bruhl and therefore to Blondel, was well aware of the danger of introducing into sociology such clear-cut dichotomies. His functionalist approach led him to discover 'useful' functions even for something as apparently pathological as crime, and consequently to introduce the abnormal into the basic structure of society. This does not mean, however, that he is in favour of a sociogenetic theory of psychic disturbance. On the contrary, he contrasts suicide, which is dependent on social factors, with mental disorder, which is the outcome of 'psycho-organic' causes. He demonstrates the lack of statistical correlation between the suicide rate and the rate of mental disorder in widely different countries. And yet it was Durkheim who gave the sociology of mental disorder a concept which is one of the most fruitful and the most widely used today, at least in the United States: anomie. There are two different definitions of anomie in Durkheim's work. They are different, but complementary: one is objective and the other is subjective. The objective definition is found in *The Division of Labour in Society*: anomie is characterized by the absence of control and therefore of stability and regularity in the relations between different social 'functions'; this results in conflict between organisms which are theoretically interdependent. The subjective definition can be found in *Suicide*: anomie is characterized by a lack of control over passions, unfettered desires, impatience with rules and regulations, irritation and disgust, according to whether the period is one of prosperity or depression. In other words, there is a repercussion within the individual consciousness of an objective phenomenon, the absence of established rules. To understand suicide it is, of course, necessary to shift one's attention from the objective aspect of anomie to the subjective, since it is only through individual consciousness that social factors can take effect. Again, however, Durkheim did not apply the concept of anomie to the study of mental disorders, since he thought they were due to purely physiological or psychological factors. It is odd, nevertheless, that French psychiatrists and sociologists did not pay more attention to the concept of anomie. It was not until it was taken up by American social scientists that it began to occupy a central position in the study of the social origins of psychic disturbance.

Roughly at the same period as Durkheim, Pierre Janet was carrying out his solitary work, which led him progressively from psychiatry to sociology. At the end of the nineteenth century and the beginning of the twentieth, therefore, we are dealing with two movements: one starting from sociology and moving towards psychiatry, the other following the opposite route, but both reaching

17

the same conclusion, which is that there is a social dimension to mental illness. Pierre Janet put forward the idea of psychic tension, which he defined in two ways: quantitatively by the amount of psychic resources, and qualitatively by the hierarchical position of the activities of which a person is capable. Thus, if a person has a constitutional 'poverty' of resources, or if he is subject to temporary exhaustion caused, for example, by having to take an examination or by family conflicts and problems, then his tension is lowered.[4] Already we have here the beginnings of a sociogenetic theory, at least in relation to certain illnesses, such as psychasthenia. Janet also points out that present-day society demands of us an ever-increasing expenditure of psychic energy. We can no longer predict the reactions even of our relatives and close friends: things are changing rapidly and a heightened tension is required to adjust our behaviour to the elements in our situation which are new to us. Our civilization is an exhausting one. The mentally-ill person, lacking in psychic resources, either takes refuge in solitude or, like 'Madeleine', creates a phantasy world where imaginary people behave exactly according to his wishes.[5] We need not describe at greater length the clinical data Janet collected to show how this lowering of tension brings about a loss of the higher mental functions (perception, speech, attention, memory, etc.) and the development of secondary phenomena (agitation, automatism, etc.). The important thing about Janet's theory is that it explains the increase in neurosis and psychasthenia by the growing complexity of social life. So long as society does not create problems which are too difficult and does not demand too much of the individual, subjects who are disposed to psychic disorders can succeed in adapting and in leading a normal existence; this is what happens in homogeneous and traditional communities, such as rural communities. But in the progressive and heterogeneous modern city competition and the struggle for higher economic and social status lead us rapidly to burn up our last resources.

3 Marxism and mental illness

The second main current of sociological thought to provide a basis for a sociology of mental illness is Marxism.

With Marxism we are dealing with two tendencies. The first uses the concepts of class struggle and alienation to bring to light the pathogenic effect of economic conditions. The second, represented by orthodox Soviet psychiatry, is based on Pavlov's theory of conditioned responses. As an example of the first tendency, let us take the French Marxist, Le Guillant.[6] He does not consider that an explanation of mental disorder by bad living conditions, such as

18

slums, low wages, unemployment or drunkenness, is a Marxist explanation. Although the effect of such factors on individuals is undeniable, to create a causal link between these factors and reactive psychosis would obviously be an over-simplification. Social influences must be apprehended within the wider context of the contradictions of capitalist society and their impact on individual consciousness. Marxist dialectics prove that all phenomena in any natural sphere (and consequently the phenomenon of abnormality) must necessarily be observed in their environmental context. But our view of the environment must not be shortsighted and obsessed with detail; it must take into account the total real situation and the divisions and contradictions of society. The explanation does not lie in accidents, however spectacular, such as wars, revolutions or strikes, but in technical, material or spiritual transformations which create difficult or insoluble problems for man. Pathogenic conflicts in the individual are the repercussion or reflection of the general conflicts of capitalist society. It should also be noted that Le Guillant takes into account spiritual change as well as material change. Basing himself on a quotation from Mao Tse-tung, he states that one must consider not only the relations of production and the conflict between the forces of production, although these are fundamental, but also the whole complex of attendant contradictions of an ideological, political and cultural nature.

Therefore, the first task of psychotherapy is to change the social environment and improve the conditions of life. Leaving aside psychosis, in which social disturbances play only a secondary role, neurosis should disappear with the transition from a capitalist to a communist society, since the latter abolishes the contradictions of the former. It does, in fact, seem as if neurosis has disappeared from Soviet society, until we realize that it does not appear in mental-health statistics because it is now treated in general instead of psychiatric hospitals. This indicates that there has been an actual displacement of neurotic symptoms from the psychic to the somatic field, conflicts being expressed through organic disturbances. We thus come to a new dimension in the study of mental disorder which is cultural and not purely sociological; we shall return to it later.

Soviet psychiatry is, of course, based on Pavlovian theory. Does this imply a paradoxical rejection of Marxism as a sociological doctrine in favour of a return to a purely organismic conception of mental illness? This is the opinion of a number of Marxists, such as Gabel: 'We are faced with a paradox which is difficult to evade if we persist in seeing Pavlovian theory as the essential basis of Marxist psychiatry. Man's normal consciousness is determined by his social existence, whereas morbid consciousness is extra-social

19

and depends on the influence of essentially biological factors.'[7] This is very close to Charles Blondel's conception, the paradoxical nature of which we pointed out earlier. But let us not go too fast: we must realize that Pavlov, in drawing attention to the responses of feeding and self-defence, also emphasizes the importance of rational and social elements. He recognizes that in animals who are given experimental neuroses, and even more so in humans, if two reflexes are conditioned in a particular way, a conflict can result which inhibits them both. He is thus recognizing the importance of conditioning, and consequently the influence of society. He then points out that this conditioning becomes more complex as one progresses from animals to man, because of the appearance of speech, culture and ethical values. Thus Pavlov is also finally led to sociology: mental illness is caused either by congenital deficiency or by the impact of an environment which is threatening to the individual, exhausts his nervous energy, inhibits the functioning of the central nervous system and thus liberates the subcortical or neuro-vegetative functions. The appropriate therapy is sociological rather than biological, as would have been the case if Pavlov's theory were merely 'organismic'. The central nervous system must be strengthened by creating an environment where the individual feels secure. On the other hand, by improving the conditioning of the feeding and self-defence responses, it becomes easier to channel the sexual response so that it can be sublimated into social feelings.[8]

The Pavlovian approach and the sociological approach are not contradictory. They constitute different tendencies, but they can be complementary. However, Marxism is far from being totally represented by the two schools of thought we have briefly examined. We mentioned Gabel: he was not satisfied with the sociological explanations derived from Marx because he felt they were oversimplifications, nor with Pavlovian theory, which seemed to him a return to organicism. He criticized both schools for ignoring the dialectical explanation, which was Marx's great discovery, in favour of mechanistic explanations. In fact, he found the work of Binswanger, in spite of its idealistic terminology, much closer to Marxism than what is known as Marxist psychiatry, because it offers so many concrete examples of 'delirious thought' determined by the being. 'When Binswanger speaks of the dialectical unity of the self and the world, when he evokes "the close functional correlativity between Gnosis and Praxis", or generally emphasizes the importance of Praxis, it is hard to distinguish his thinking from true Marxism.' The task which Gabel undertakes is to find a definition of social alienation which would empirically encompass at least one form of psychiatric alienation: schizophrenia. He thinks the formula can be found in Lukacs's definition of ideology and false consciousness, interpreted as a breakdown in the dialectical grasp of reality, or reification. This breakdown in dialectical perception and this reification are related to the morbid rationalization characteristic of schizophrenia. Basing himself on the work of Minkowski and other psychiatrists, Gabel defines schizophrenic thinking as the spacialization of duration, the fragmentation of wholes, a logic of pure identity. In other words, Marxism, in that it is a theory of false consciousness, is essentially a critical theory of a form of delirious thought; what is more, it provides 'a terminology which is well-worn by a semisecular critique of an ideological critique'.[9]

We will not venture into the other aspect of Gabel's theory, which is complementary to the first, and consists of interpreting political ideologies in terms of schizophrenic thought. Let us simply make the following points:

(1) Gabel's sociology is only applicable to schizophrenia; it does not cover other disorders, such as, for example, paranoia.

(2) He does not *a priori* reject organic pathogenesis: 'dialectical thinking being an arduous intellectual process, it is permissible to assume that the self which is weakened by an organic cause will, in its psychological grasp of reality, take refuge in the comfort of non-dialectical thinking'.[10]

(3) Finally and most important, if we have understood him right, he orients Marxist sociology away from a sociogenetic theory and towards the sociological description of morbid structures, both social and individual.

Gabel's theory is, of course, open to criticism (his comparison of phenomena of social pathology with schizophrenia, his interpretation of schizophrenia, etc.). But what is of interest to us, in terms of the theory of ideas, is this mutation of Marxist sociology from a sociogenetic theory to structuralism.

4 Psychoanalysis

Psychoanalysis has made an important contribution, both to psychiatry and to sociology.[11] Its influence on psychiatry is outside our present scope, and we have devoted a whole book to psychoanalysis and sociology. The only question we shall deal with in this section is whether psychoanalysis, through its sociological extensions, has an original theory to contribute in the particular field of the sociology of mental disorder. At first sight it appears that the answer is in the negative. First of all because Freud, contrary to the Marxists we have just been studying, discounts the role of socio-economic factors, in particular the class struggle, and gives the critical role to biological and especially sexual factors. It is true that later on, when anthropologists cast doubts on the universality of the Oedipus complex, there was some attempt to introduce a cultural element into the interpretations of psychoanalysis.[12] (Roheim protested, pointing out that the Oedipus complex is a universal biological feature of the human race, due to the slow maturation of the human organism.[13]) In the second place, psychoanalysis deals with 'history', a history in which the fate of the individual is sealed in the very first years of life. This would tend towards underestimation of social factors and their influence during the course of a person's life; it would imply the replacement of sociology, which is interested in generalities, by history, which is the recording of a stream of discrete and contingent events.

Nevertheless, in other ways, psychoanalysis leads us to recognize the value of sociology:

(1) It is concerned with early experience; it takes the patient back from his present situation to his childhood, and reconstructs his relationship with his mother, father and siblings. It has therefore drawn the attention of psychiatrists and sociologists or social psychiatrists to the importance of family influences in the genesis of psychic disorders.

(2) It recognizes that these disorders are only partly caused by traumas in early childhood. This is a point which is often neglected, but which in our opinion is essential; the traumas must be reawakened by the social situation in which the individual finds himself. Thus the disturbance originates not from a single but from a double trauma. For this reason, it is essential for the psychiatrist to consider factors outside the family, and this leads him to sociological research.

(3) As psychoanalysis is a dialogue between patient and analyst, it has awakened an interest in a particular problem—a sociological problem if any, or at least a prelude to sociology: the problem of communication.

(4) Psychoanalytic theory has changed over time, the trend being towards a much more sociological approach. Karen Horney noted as early as 1939 in *New Ways in Psychoanalysis*: 'A prevailing sociological orientation ... takes the place of a prevailing anatomical-physiological one.' In insisting more on the defence mechanisms than on the libido, contemporary psychoanalysis gives more importance to sociology than the older school.

It is therefore not surprising that the sociology of mental illness often makes use of the techniques, theoretical suggestions and vocabulary of psychoanalysis. We believe that this was first of all an antidote to the over-use of statistics—sociologists were reminded of the importance of the case history, of the necessity of complementing a positivistic sociology by a *verstehen* approach. It even had the beneficial effect of refining statistical methods, as we shall see in the next chapter. It forced the statistician to reintroduce into his calculations a variable which he had often neglected, the influence of the family. In the second place, it had the effect of liberating psychiatry from such typologies as Kraepelin's; in fact, this created a certain amount of confusion among sociologists studying mental illness, as they were used to establishing correlations between a particular type of illness and a particular social factor. It oriented psychiatry towards a more dynamic perspective, uniting the organic with the symbolic functioning of the personality. Freudian theory has, of course, contributed many new ideas to the understanding of this symbolic functioning. Besides these methodological contributions, there are also linguistic ones, i.e. the introduction into the vocabulary of sociology of so many words and concepts which are so familiar that their origin is often forgotten: inferiority complex, frustration, scapegoat, psychic conflict, rationalization, repression, catharsis, sublimation, resistence, transference.

It is, of course, impossible to list all the research in the sociology of mental disorder that has used techniques, vocabulary or theoretical suggestions drawn from psychoanalysis; we shall come across some examples in the pages that follow. However, it is worth pointing out, as Parsons did, that divergence from social norms which distinguishes the mentally-ill person can occur at three different levels: the family level, the community level, and the level of society as a whole. Since norms are always internalized through the intermediary of small groups, such as neighbourhoods or families, the psychoanalyst always tends, even when taking a broad social viewpoint, to look for the primary causes of disorientation within the family. Either the child internalizes already disoriented parents or else family conflicts will be the cause of his disorientation.[14]

In spite of these undeniable contributions, the sociologist interested in psychiatry can only accept psychoanalytic theory if he reminds the psychoanalyst that he is interested only in one aspect of the question. Family experience is important, but one must not forget that economic and social forces impinge on the family and therefore on the family experience of the child. This is in fact a dialectical process; the sociologist studying mental illness must be aware of its constant two-way action. To give a few examples: the widow who is forced to work and neglects her child; the Negro mother who prefers her light-skinned child to her darker child because he is closer to the Aryan ideal that society has conditioned her to accept; the unemployed father who hinders his son's super-ego formation because of his own degrading situation; wives working in factories because of the myth of national productivity. All these cases and many more are social and not just family phenomena.[15]

Psychoanalysis drew the sociologist's attention to the importance of the socialization process in the first years of life. However, the sociologist noticed that child-care practices vary according to the social group, that there is a difference between country- and city-dwellers and, within the city, between working-class and middle-class families: each class has its own sub-culture. Whereas before we were led from early experience to society, we now make the transition from family experience to the sociology of groups.

Before ending this section, we need to say something of the extension of psychoanalysis known as 'socioanalysis'. It can take many different forms, ranging from the type of group analysis that was applied to cases of war trauma too numerous to be treated individually to Moreno's sociodrama and to the sociometry of the French school of M. and Mme Van Bockstaele. The first form is a situation of multiple transference which adds nothing new to the contribution psychoanalysis has made to the sociology of psychic disturbance. As for Moreno, he was dealing with the social adjustment, not only of the individual to the group, but also—which leads us directly into sociology—with the adjustment of groups to each other. The real subject in sociodrama is the sick group, with its internal problems, confronting another group composed of the therapist and his ego auxiliaries, or even the public of the sociometric theatre. It can also be a group with external problems, as in the case of white versus Negro in the United States.[16] Although speech is mainly replaced by action, a situation somewhat removed from orthodox psychoanalysis, the groups acting on the stage have a 'history', and we have seen that the history-sociology conflict is one of the obstacles to the use of psychoanalytic theory by sociologists. The French Sociometric Association, which is based on group dynamics as much as on psychoanalysis, eliminates the history aspect. The two groups involved, the client group and the analyst group, are in an a-historical situation. They are constituted at a given point in time, and although they are made up of individuals with their own personal history, these histories are not taken into consideration, and the anonymity of the group hinders or prevents their introduction into interpersonal relations. Since the client group cannot talk about itself, but only about the analyst group, on which it has hardly any information, the conflict and resistances it exhibits take on a purely sociological character.[17]

5 American theories of mental disorder

In America there seem to be few equivalents of the broad systematic theories of European writers. These theories tend to be replaced by a mere accumulation of restricted empirical studies. This impression is confirmed by the fact that Americans have criticized the generalities of the Europeans for being too far removed from the facts, even though they have adopted concepts evolved by European sociologists: we alluded earlier to the popularity of the concept of anomie in the United States. But to the Americans it is not sufficient to speak in terms of anomie without also making a precise inquiry into its specific character according to time and place. The Marxist concept of alienation may be valid, but not if it is only applied to a general description of the alienated individual in a hostile world; the nature of the hostility must also be specified. In short, it is necessary to study anomie or alienation in a concrete manner by placing them in their various contexts, such as acculturation, social change and economic crisis.[18] It would be wrong, however, at least at the present time, to oppose the United States and Europe in the dichotomy between general theory and empirical research. In France at present there is also a swing towards empirical research in the sociology of mental disorder. This is really a universal movement, not one which is peculiar to America: it springs from an increasing desire to model human sciences on natural sciences, to aim, above all, for precision.

It is possible to distinguish two main periods in American 'social psychiatry'. We will only be concerned here with the facts directly related to our more narrowly defined subject. During the first period, although sociologists were not dealing with psychiatric matters, they developed a number of concepts which were later used by psychiatrists: Veblen's conspicuous consumption of the leisured classes (its imitation by the middle classes leading to tension and problems), McDougall's explanation of workers' revolts by frustration and scapegoating, etc. But sociologists were still only providing suggestions for research until Thomas, in his study of Polish peasant immigrants in the U.S.A., was able to show that the lack of social integration of immigrants in their new environment could cause delinquency and produce a higher rate of mental illness among immigrants than that of their native country. There followed a profusion of studies, not always classifiable into social psychiatry proper or the sociology of mental disorder, e.g. the work of Burrow, Kimball Young, H. Adolphus Miller, Elton Mayo, etc. In 1929 Thomas created a new section of the American Sociological Association whose importance was to develop increasingly, 'Sociology and Psychiatry'.[19]

The creation of this particular field brought together socio-logists and psychiatrists who had until then been working in isolation, even though they made use of each other's work. It greatly increased the volume of research. We shall be dealing with some of this research in the later chapters of this book. Briefly, it can be divided into three branches: the first relating to the social and cultural dimensions of mental illness, the second to social relations in therapy, and the third to prevention as a social policy, in so far as mental-hygiene practices are regarded, not as norma-tive practices, but as experiments for the testing of theoretical hypotheses.[20]

In each of these main subdivisions, and especially in the first, there have been so many studies of such a diverse and even con-tradictory nature that it may seem difficult to discern any continuity. It would be wrong, however, to see the sociology of mental dis-order as a chaos of purely empirical studies with no order to them at all: they all relate to each other in some way.

First, because they all imply the same *Gestalt* conception of mental illness: culture, social system and personality are functional variables which are interdependent and interrelated.

Second, because they are all 'conceptualized': this system of concepts links the various studies, integrates them into the total picture and enables theoretical conclusions to be drawn from concrete facts. Mme Rocheblave-Spenlé, in the chapter of her book, *La Notion de Rôle en Psychologie Sociale*, entitled 'The Concept of Role and Behaviour Disorders',[21] recently gave an ex-cellent example of how this conceptualization integrates widely different studies. In order to understand this chapter it is important to remember that the idea of role refers us to two other concepts. The first is the *social norm*, where the person's role is the behaviour pattern which other people expect of him, and which conforms to the rules of social life. The second is *communication*, where the role is the code used to decipher the flood of messages received, dis-tortions occurring whenever the decoding system used by the re-ceiver is not tuned in to the transmitter's code. Social norms in turn refer us to the collective value system. This means that finally the sociology of mental disorder uses a 'reference system' of four terms: role, norm, value and communication. Some writers, such as Cameron, will make much more use of the concepts of role and norm with reference to the roles of the mentally ill, which represent, in the same way as normal roles, the individual's response to others, his attempts to adjust to reality, and the equivalent of 'relatively fixed and crystallized models . . . of behaviour'.[22] Others place more importance on collective values: Karen Horney, for example, feels that the origin of neurosis lies in the conflict between our ideology, with its emphasis on fellowship and the high value it places on sacrifice, and the norms of a capitalist society based on economic competition and the struggle for social status. This conflict of values is, of course, also a conflict of roles, the same individual having to play contradictory roles, some of which are acquired in the family and others imposed by social competition. His conflict is the internalization of the external conflict of social roles.[23] Yet others stress difficulties of communication. For example, this is how Mme Rocheblave-Spenlé summarizes Newcomb's theory.[24]

> The psychotic generally thinks that others perceive what he
> wants to communicate. If he is impersonating the President of
> the United States, he believes that his status is recognized
> by others and that his actions are in accordance with accepted
> norms. But as the position he has assumed does not correspond
> to reality and others do not share his beliefs, his role-appropriate
> actions do not have a communicative function and have the
> effect of excluding him from the community. He is convinced,
> however, that the break in communication is due to the other
> person, who is not receiving his messages adequately and
> does not send him back properly formulated ones; in short,
> he accuses the other of being mad. Moreover, when
> communication between two people is disrupted, it is often
> difficult at first sight to establish which of the two is insane.

To distinguish the mad person from the sane person it is necessary to base oneself on an external criterion: the concordance of the sane person's behaviour with that of the group.[25]

Thus the reference system of sociology provides the various empirical studies with a common fund of concepts which holds out the promise of a future synthesis. This is not to say that general theories have not yet been developed in the United States. Some of them are not very fruitful compared with European theories. When Leighton states that there is more mental disorder in disintegrated than in integrated sectors of society, he is only restating Comte's theory, which we described at the beginning of this chapter. However, he is trying to make it more precise by proposing a dual index of phenomena defining social disintegration, and by distinguishing three processes of disintegration: on the technical level rapid changes in technology, on the social level mobility, and on the level of ideology or value-systems the conflict between these systems. In other words, he does not limit himself to a general idea; he breaks it down into components to come nearer to the concrete approach of social psychiatrists. He also introduces an important qualification: without the existence of

27

morbid predisposition, social disintegration does not necessarily bring about individual disintegration, but social disintegration does contribute to mental illness by the physical damage it can do to the individual (greater frequency of traumas, infections, inadequate diet, etc.) or by its genetic impact (the socio-cultural environment can affect heredity through sexual relations).[26]

We will not attempt a review of all the theories of American social psychiatrists, but two authors are worthy of mention, as they are among the most influential in our field and happen to be the founders of a thriving school of thought: a psychiatrist, Sullivan, and a sociologist, Parsons.

Sullivan[27] saw the individual, not as an isolated being equipped with given instincts and drives, but as a social being to whom society continually presents problems. The self to Sullivan is the equivalent of the electron to the physicist. The physicist is interested only in constellations of electrons, not in the electron itself; in the same way, the psychiatrist must study, not individuals, but interpersonal situations. When I define myself it is always in relation to others, as an American, as a member of Western culture, as part of industrial society, etc. If I were a Negro, I would define myself differently. I am only the meeting-place of my body with its physical environment, of my psyche with other psyches. The individual has two goals: the satisfaction of physical needs, a biological necessity, and security, a cultural necessity. Both are in fact linked, as the cultural *milieu* may condemn certain biological satisfactions, such as sexual satisfaction, and the need for security includes or integrates biological satisfaction. However, neurosis is mainly related to insecurity, and since security depends on acceptance or rejection by the social environment, neurosis can be defined as a disturbance in human relations. This conclusion carries two consequences. The most important thing for the psychiatrist is not the study of society as a whole, its organization into classes or castes, but the study of formative relationships, of the way in which socialization takes place in the formative years. (It is understood that for Sullivan these years do not end, as in the case of psychoanalysis, with the resolution of the Oedipus complex, but continue throughout adolescence.) Therapy will therefore consist in re-establishing the severed communication and restructuring relationships. In the second place—and this is, in our opinion, the most subtle part of Sullivan's analysis—psychiatric observation is not a purely objective observation where the doctor steps outside himself to describe a foreign being; it is like any other interactive situation, it embraces both the patient's behaviour and the experience of the observer. Sullivan had a very great influence on American psychiatry, and a whole school developed around him.[28]

One must admit that from the sociological point of view this approach cannot lead very far as it presupposes a certain sociological nominalism, even if only in the field of interpersonal relations.

Parsons, on the other hand, is a sociologist, and one of the most respected and widely followed in the United States; at the same time he has taken a great deal of interest in medical problems and in psychiatry. We shall therefore close this account of the main theories of psychiatric sociology with a review of some of his theories.[29] Our starting-point will be the theory of 'deviance', a term which describes all behaviour deviating from that prescribed by society, as opposed to conformist behaviour, which makes social life possible. Parsons classifies phenomena of deviance along two axes. The first axis is conformity—alienation, with at one extreme escape from society, and at the other over-conformist behaviour and rigidity in the application of norms. The second is passivity—activity, with at one end insensitivity to social sanctions, which places the individual on the margin of society (tramps), and at the other acts of open rebellion. It is possible to fit a theory of mental disorder into the sociological theory of deviance. In mental disorder there is divergence between the behaviour of the individual and the expectations of others, between actual behaviour and social norms. Although the psychiatrist studies individual cases of divergence, the conflict he is concerned with is an internalized one. Therefore it comes from outside the individual, and necessarily refers the psychiatrist back to the sociologist. The structure of the personality is only a reflection in the individual of the social structure. Parsons distinguishes three types of individual: (1) the personality system is idiosyncratic in relation to the social system; (2) the individual is so engulfed by society that his own personality is destroyed (which is the case in all compulsive, phobic and anxious states); (3) the social system is disorganized and the sick person internalizes this disorganization. The unifying and integrating forces in social systems are their 'value orientations'; these value orientations constitute one of the main themes of Parsons' sociology. Thus sociology actually provides a framework for the study of mental disorder.

In any action we are faced with dilemmas and we are compelled to make a choice. Value orientations are 'variables', which serve to describe our actions. The first variable is the dilemma of *universalism* versus *particularism*. In urban industrial societies there can be a conflict between family roles, such as father or wife, and occupational roles, which are more particularistic. One example is the conflict between the affective ties of the family and the formal ties of bureaucratic structures; it is no accident that

bureaucratic organizations produce so many cases of mental disorder. The second variable is the *affectivity—neutrality* dilemma.
The conflict here is between the emotionally loaded roles which
shape the personality in early life and the neutral roles encountered
after adolescence. The third variable is the dilemma of *collectivity-
orientation* versus *self-orientation*: in our industrial society, when
the individual cannot reconcile the demands of the community
with his personal needs psychic disturbance soon occurs. This would
explain why there is more mental illness in certain sectors of the
population than in others. *Gratification—deprivation* gives us a
fourth variable: if we carry out our roles properly, it is because
there is some advantage in doing so—enjoyment, economic success,
a rise in status. There may, however, be some needs which are not
met in a given social system, which is why it is necessary to include the problem of frustration in any sociological study of
mental illness. The last variable is the dimension of *diffuseness*
versus *specificity* of roles. Durkheim's theory of anomie gives an
excellent example of specificity: the available roles can only absorb
a small part of the personality, the personality system becomes
blocked, with repercussions on the mental health of the individual.

If mental pathology is to have a place in a sociological theory
of deviance, correspondingly psychotherapy must be included in a
sociological theory of social control, since the function of psychotherapy is to reintegrate the mentally ill into the social system. On
one hand, psychotherapy is part of a wider system of control
mechanisms and therefore comes into the field of general sociology.
On the other hand, society puts pressure on the sick person
through the intermediary of the psychiatrist; the sociologist must
try to encompass all the latent mechanisms which check deviance
and re-establish the balance between society and the individual.
'Deliberate psychotherapy is . . . only the part of the iceberg which
extends above the water. The considerably larger part is that below
the surface of the water. Even its existence has been largely unknown to most psychiatrists.'[30] This is why the contributions of
sociology are so essential.

6 The choice

Can we draw any conclusions from this long historical survey?
Fundamentally, we have been dealing with two sets of theories.
The first start with psychiatry and progress towards sociology:
Morel, psychoanalysis, Sullivan. The second begin with sociology
and move towards psychiatry: Audiffrend via Comte, Blondel via
Lévy-Bruhl, Le Guillant via Marx, to quote only a few. But in
both cases we are dealing with a sociologist's sociology, and it is

worth asking whether this is a good situation, or whether it would not be more suitable for psychiatrists to produce their own sociology, instead of tending towards or borrowing from a sociology outside their field.[31]

Moreover, these theories are struggling with a double difficulty represented by their extreme generality on the one hand and their specificity on the other. They are too specific in the sense that they highlight only one factor, such as disorganization, anomie, communication difficulties, conflicts of values or of roles. Parsons is perhaps the only author who has tried to take into account the multiplicity of factors by reducing them to a series of miscellaneous examples. But these different theories ultimately tend towards a sociogenetic approach (even if they are interested in the physical aspect of illness). This is where their second aspect comes in: they are excessively general. A distinction must obviously be made (even after eliminating lesions or infections) between neurosis and psychosis. To speak of social factors in mental disorder in general does not mean very much. The arguments we have outlined in this chapter are certainly valid for neurosis, but to what extent do they apply to psychosis? A whole new set of problems are raised at the end of this historical review: we have to choose between a single-factor interpretation and the acceptance of a multiplicity of factors, between a sociogenetic and a structuralist approach. We shall tackle these problems gradually in the chapters that follow.

II Methodological problems

1 Three disciplines distinguished

As empirical studies became more and more numerous, what was required of sociology was more a body of operational concepts than a set of guide-lines; the emphasis shifted from problems of theory to the problems of perfecting techniques of investigation. Method was gaining ascendancy over system.

From the methodological point of view, it seems feasible to make a distinction between the three disciplines we enumerated in our Introduction: social psychiatry, based on the case study; the sociology of mental disorder, based on the statistical method; and ethnopsychiatry, based on the cross-cultural method. We would thus only need to deal in this chapter with techniques of statistical investigation. But some psychiatrists claim that statistics are of little use to them, that social science concepts have to be broken down to become meaningful in research; the personality-environment relationship has to be split into a series of relations between one specific individual and a given environment, and only the psychiatrist is competent to do this. They are focusing on the very conflict we detected earlier between the sociology of mental illness and sociology proper. This is in fact a conflict between two methods, statistics and the case study. One should not conclude that statistics have no value, but only that they have no value in social psychiatry in the strictest sense. Case studies are concerned only with individuals, and no matter how many individual cases are collected, they will never constitute a meaningful pattern. A mentally-ill person can be explained, but mental illness cannot; only the statistician is able to detect meaningful patterns. Although our sociology of mental illness survives the criticism of the psychiatrists, this criticism does have a point: it reveals that each science has its own particular method. We could say the same about the comparative method: it will obviously be the one used by ethnopsychiatry, as the object here is to detect variations in the frequency or symptomatology of mental illness among a multiplicity of civilizations. The sociology of mental illness, on the other hand, is concerned with our own society and with situations where the psychiatrist and the patient share the same value system. In the main it is true to say that each science chooses its own method, but in reality things are more complex than this. In the present chapter we shall see that even within the framework of the sociology of mental disorder many other methods of investigation can be used besides the statistical method.

2 The statistical method

Because this method is fundamental to our work, we shall begin with it. It has in fact been strongly criticized, but the criticism, as we shall see, bears more on its application than on its validity as a basic method for the sociological study of mental illness. The transition from the essentially psychological approach of social psychiatry to the sociological approach necessarily requires that we change from case studies to the study of groups. No scientist to my knowledge has ever complained of this progression from the microscopic to the macroscopic level, which opens up new perspectives to the investigator. Durkheim showed that suicide followed sociological regularities which could not be analysed in terms of psychopathological categories. Even though each suicide can be traced back to certain conditions particular to the individual, it is still related on the macroscopic level to other phenomena which only sociology can detect with the aid of statistics. In geology the laws governing the behaviour of sandbanks are not derived from the kinematics or dynamics of one grain of sand, and in biology the laws of evolution emerge on a different plane from the genetic processes which explain mutations. The sociology of mental illness cannot be a synthesis of all the conclusions reached previously by social psychiatrists, for even if social psychiatry were a fully developed science it would still only be microscopic in its approach and could not give us information on a level other than that of the individual. Macroscopic observation can disregard the individual components, since the patterns it discovers are on another scale and are not the result of a mere sum of parts. Clearly, the only way to avoid perpetual extrapolations from the results of social psychiatry to sociology is to make a 'methodological leap' to a position where the use of statistics will enable sociological laws to emerge which cannot be perceived at a lower level. According to

Heisenberg's principle, if the attention is focused at a certain level it is not possible to see phenomena belonging to another observational level: 'It is impossible to focus at the same time on two levels if their order of magnitude differs too much. . . . Whatever one gains in precision at one level one loses at another.'[1] This discrepancy between two observational viewpoints and the fact that in all scientific fields—physics, biology, etc.—different regularities can emerge on a macroscopic level which cannot be extracted by analysis from microscopic regularities justify the statistical method as a basis for the sociology of mental illness. We have remained so far on a theoretical plane. In practice the statistical study of mental illness is fraught with problems. We will review them shortly. However, since the use of statistics is theoretically justified, these problems have but one solution: the progressive refinement of statistical methods and not, as some social psychiatrists would like, their wholesale rejection.

We can go even further than this. It is known that many explanations have been put forward for mental disorder in other fields besides social psychiatry. Some emphasize social factors and others hereditary metabolic disturbance or the abnormal production of diamines; others see mental illness as a form of encephalopathy, and yet others attribute disturbances of thought to biochemical changes in the cerebral tissue. We can set all these theories aside exactly as Durkheim set aside the link between suicide and psychopathology. As we have seen, what is true at one level can cease to be true at another. Tuberculosis and syphilis are organic diseases, yet no doctor complains of statistical surveys conducted by health services to discover which sectors of the population are most affected by these illnesses, or to follow, on a macroscopic level, the progress of the fight to eradicate them. The sociology of mental illness can therefore ignore the causes of mental disturbance, whether organic or social, and see whether, from a higher vantage-point, it is not possible to detect certain patterns that go unnoticed at a lower level. These patterns can then only be of a sociological order, even if at a more basic level the patterns emerging are biochemical, genetic or anatomic.

Statisticians in the social sciences use a certain number of measures which we must first briefly define:

(1) The *rate of incidence* of mental disorder, which measures the frequency of appearance of new cases (only first admissions to hospital are counted, readmissions being classified separately) during a stated interval, usually one year.

(2) The *rate of prevalence*, which measures the total number of patients during a given interval of time (those entering hospital during the interval and leaving before the end of the interval, those

entering during the interval and remaining in treatment, those in hospital long before the interval in question and remaining there at the end of the interval, and those, finally, who were in hospital when the interval began and who were discharged before it ended). If one then adds to the patients in public or private institutions people who are ill, but do not seek treatment, one obtains the true rate of prevalence, whereas the previous definition is the rate of prevalence of treated mental disorder.

(3 The *rate of illness during a lifetime* used by Scandinavian psychiatrists, which also includes all persons affected by psychosis who have returned to normal life, since these psychiatrists do not believe that psychosis can be cured.

(4) Finally, the *predicted rate*, which predicts the number of people in a given population who will fall ill within their lifetime.[2] Obviously, this percentage depends on the life-expectation at various ages of the population in question, which must be taken into account in making the calculation.

With the exception of a small number of psychiatrists who were interested in the distribution of mental illness according to social or ethnic group, such as Kraepelin,[3] it was not until 1930 that statistical studies really developed universally. Unfortunately, these studies are not always comparable because of differences in the way the information was gathered and processed.[4] It is true that this is more of a past than a future difficulty, since one can hope that international organizations will be able to impose common norms on research workers everywhere, so that data may be compared. But there is another more serious obstacle. Between the raw data and their processing the psychiatrist's classification inevitably intervenes, varying according to the period and the country. For example, the French include epilepsy among mental disorders, while the Americans do not; on the other hand, the Americans make schizophrenia cover a much wider field than the French, which means that the same term is applied to two different nosological entities. To a certain extent this obstacle too can be overcome by a preliminary definition of the terms used, e.g. by defining the criteria of schizophrenia for a particular study.[5] But a more serious problem is that the research worker intervenes personally with his ideologies, the habits he has acquired during his training and the assumptions of the particular school to which he belongs.[6] Lapouse suggests that one of the reasons for the high rate of psychosis in the lower social classes is that psychiatrists are reluctant to label their upper-class patients psychotic.[7] When the author was collecting data in the hospitals of Rio de Janeiro, he was hindered by the fact that at different times of day there were different psychiatrists on duty, each with his own way of perceiving

35

and classifying disorders, so that patients might receive different diagnoses, although inspection of their files showed their disorders to be similar.

Apart from these difficulties, statistical techniques are progressively becoming more refined, which gives us a reasonable hope of developing a sociology of mental disorder. Let us give two examples. The first derives from the frequently made statement that, with the exception of periods of war, the rate of mental illness is steadily increasing. In the U.S.A. it is observed to have jumped from 204·2 per 100,000 population in 1910 to 335·3 in 1936. How meaningful are these figures? Deutsch suggested that the reason why there are more mentally-ill people is that there are more hospitals: growth in the number of people treated keeps pace with the increase in the number of beds available.[8] People tend to be more concerned about their health than before. Society's conception of mental illness has also changed (it is no longer to the same extent considered incurable, nor as a stigma on the family of the sick person).[9] The problem has to be considered anew. This is what Goldhamer and Marshall did in their study of psychosis. They looked at first admissions to public hospitals and private nursing-homes in Massachusetts from 1840 to 1940.[10] Several corrections had to be made: the oldest figures were inflated by the inclusion among psychotics of mental defectives, neurotics, epileptics and alcoholics; on the other hand, the present-day figures had to be corrected for senile psychosis, due to the increase in the average life-span over the last 100 years. The population of Massachusetts has also increased, and this had to be taken into account by calculating the rate of psychosis in relation to the existing population at a given date. The result of these corrections was to show that the rate of psychosis had remained virtually stable throughout the whole period in question. This was in spite of profound changes in social structure over the century (disproving the theories of some social psychiatrists) and in spite of changes in the conception of health and the improvement in hospital conditions (disproving Deutsch's argument).

Despite these findings, if we are dealing with a heterogeneous population it is necessary to consider the attitudes of the community to mental illness. A recent study made in French Canada showed that the Anglo-Saxons willingly send their sick to hospital or to be treated by a psychiatrist. French Canadians, who believe that illness is an act of God, tend to keep patients at home (unless they are actually dangerous), while the Irish, who consider illness to be caused by sin, tend to hide the sick person.[11] The rate of incidence is thus affected by the general attitudes of the cultural and ethnic *milieu* towards 'insanity'. Texans of Spanish origin have a lower rate of mental disorder than Anglo-Saxon Americans (40 for men and 45 for women versus 73 and 87 respectively per 100,000 population). Could this not be because the two groups have different attitudes towards mental illness, the first preferring to look after their sick themselves and the second to have them cared for in specialized institutions?[12] It has also been found that within a homogeneous community in which attitudes are uniform, other

Diagram 1 Increase of hospitalization rates for the mentally ill

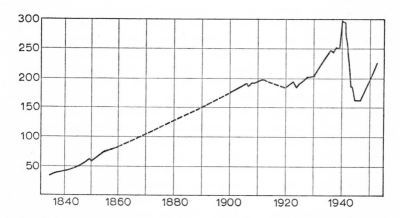

(Extracted from Henri Duchêne, 'Aspect demographique', in *Esprit*, No. 12 (December 1952), p. 878.)

factors can come into play, causing variations in rates of incidence —such as, distance from the nearest hospital, transport facilities, or simply rumours about the sort of treatment one gets at the hospital, how good the psychiatrists are or even how clean the place looks.

Another difficulty is that studies of the rate of first admissions to public and private institutions are generally limited to one state of the U.S.A. or one town. The mobility of the population can distort data collected in this way. The 1960 report of the National Institute of Mental Health gives a distribution of rates per 100,000 population ranging from 70·7 for Missouri to 938·6 for the District of Columbia; it is probable that the high figure for the District of Columbia is due to the fact that its hospital facilities attract patients from other states. Corrections are also needed here. The patients'

37

files can often provide information on mobility, but it is not always easy to keep the necessary checks. We encountered this difficulty personally in our study of mental disorder among West Indians in France. We could not accept a first admission in France as the patient's first contact with a hospital: obviously many West Indians had been treated in their native country, but exactly how many? It is difficult to tell when the only information is a statement from the patient, who may well be hiding a previous breakdown.

These numerous difficulties have led psychiatrists to replace the crude rate of incidence or prevalence of treated mental illness with the true rate of prevalence. This means not only finding out about people who have had contact with hospitals, but also about the others. One method, used by Brugger and also by Strömgren, is to question general practitioners, school-teachers and clergymen about mentally-ill people in their community who are not receiving hospital treatment.[13] This reveals many cases of disturbance that have eluded the statistical records. It is also possible to use Klemperer's method, which consists in collecting the names of 1,000 people in a particular area born within a given period, and in finding out which ones have not become mentally ill. This is a better method, in that, once the sample has been selected, the psychiatrist makes a personal visit to each home. It is not always easy, however, to locate the subjects (Klemperer only managed to trace 70 per cent of his sample.[14]) Nevertheless, the results obtained by this method are interesting. For example, Fremming, who applied it to the island of Bornholm, where he visited about 2,000 people out of the 5,500 born between 1883 and 1887, found that 15 per cent of the sample were psychotic, whereas only 3 per cent of them were in hospital.[15] Another approach is to submit all military conscripts to a neuro-psychiatric examination: this was done in the U.S.A. during the last war (induction statistic method), but, of course, it is limited to the population of an age to do their military service.[16]

The ideal situation would be to take a very small homogeneous group where the psychiatrist could visit every home. This is a method Eaton and Weil used in their brilliant study of the Hutterites.[17] But it is only rarely possible. Moreover, there is always a great danger that investigators studying small communities will consider them representative of a larger community and generalize from the results of one study to a whole area. A type of study which is becoming more and more popular is the giant interdisciplinary study involving impressive numbers of specialists, e.g. the Stirling County Project or the Midtown Mental Health Study. The technique of sampling comes into its own here, and there are signs that it will increasingly become the basis for the sociological study of mental disorder.

A second example of methodological refinement is the control of variables. If we wish to make a comparison between different populations, we need first to standardize them. For example, the proportion of men to women and of old to young people varies from one population to another. As the rate of mental disorder is dependent both on sex and age, we must make the necessary corrections to avoid being led into gross errors in our conclusions. Hollingshead and Redlich's study is a good example of the use of correction techniques.[18] However, age and sex are not the only variables. There are also differences in race, ethnic group, religion, education, living conditions and social class. These variables are interwoven. How do we decide which ones are basic and which are secondary? There is a risk, according to the orientation of the study (whether, for example, it is primarily concerned with ecological, economic or religious factors), of giving too much weight to a secondary variable and neglecting a basic one. A good example of this is given by Mehl. Many immigrants to the U.S.A. are from Catholic countries, and at least in the first generation, tend to belong to the lower social classes. The sociologist who is interested in the variable of religion is likely to state that Catholics have a higher rate of schizophrenia than Unitarians. But he needs to beware of attributing to religion what may only be the reflection of a difference in social conditions between working-class Catholics and middle-class Unitarians.[19] The sociologist must therefore substitute what could be called the 'synthetic method' for the analytical method, which consists in examining each variable separately. For example, Hollingshead and Redlich suggest two dimensions, one vertical (race, religion, ethnic membership), the other horizontal (occupation, education, residence), which are then combined to form a highly compartmentalized structure. Individuals can then be categorized according to their positions on both axes.[20]

In our opinion this 'structuring' of variables represents an enormous progress relative to previous analytical studies; but as research techniques become more refined, they also grow in complexity, and the social scientist needs to work in closer collaboration with the statistician.

Another way of controlling variables is, of course, to set up an experimental group and a control group. For example, among New York Puerto Ricans, one forms two groups with the same sex ratio, average age, number of single people, average family size, number of Catholics and number of owner-occupiers. The economic status of the two groups is then controlled, the mean value of the properties being $7,800 in the experimental group and $6,500 in the control group. The family income is $2,010 for the experimental group and $2,680 for the control group. But this method need not detain us, as it is common both to the sociology of mental illness and to other branches of sociology.

3 The case-study method

Whereas the statistical method is fundamental to sociology, the case-study method forms the basis of social psychiatry. This means, of course, that it is of less relevance in sociology than in social psychiatry, either in the strictest sense or a branch social psychology. However, as we shall see, it can undoubtedly be of value to the sociologist.

We shall not attempt to describe and criticize the case-study approach, but we shall remind the reader of the following points: (1) There is a choice of two methods. The first method is the questionnaire administered to mental patients or their relatives, comprising questions on organic, physical and physiological factors, on the patients' environment, and on the interaction between organic and environmental factors. This is the classical psychiatric approach.[21] The second method is more refined and probing: it is not content with the immediate responses of the subject, but delves into the 'hidden' areas, the depths of the personality, by dream interpretation and the technique of free association. (2) There are difficulties encountered by the case-study method which make it no more desirable than other methods, whatever the opinion of some investigators. First of all, what constitutes a 'case'? What differentiates a sane person from an insane person? Here the psychiatrist introduces his own conception of normal and pathological into his observations.[22] We shall return to this fundamental question later. In the second place, whereas in a statistical study the data are conducive to a certain neutrality and can form a barrier to the preconceptions of the investigator, in case studies there is an intimate relationship between the observer and the observed: the psychiatrist brings to his investigations his own personal inclinations and ideologies, his conception of reality and his past experiences. His observations become interpretations. This is why the psychoanalyst has to undergo a training analysis; it is an attempt to correct the unconscious manipulation by the psychiatrist of the subject of his analysis.

Our aim in this book is not to devise a methodology (which would quickly become a deontology) of the case study, but only to discover its possible role in the sociological study of mental illness. It appears that we may find an answer to our question in the distinction between positivist sociology and the *verstehen* approach. In the first part of this chapter we tried to see things from the point of view of Durkheimian sociology. Durkheim is concerned with *whys* and not with *hows*; he explains, but does not try to understand. Understanding would necessarily introduce psychology, since it is only possible with reference to personal experience. But since Dilthey, and especially Weber, the *verstehen* approach has become more widely accepted and has begun to undermine the bastion of psychiatry. Statistics can show correlations between particular morbid phenomena and social variables, but it cannot help us to understand these phenomena. The case-study method could therefore constitute a second branch of our sociology corresponding to the *verstehen* conception in sociology.

But unfortunately this is not the case. We may be able to understand that a man becomes depressed because his wife has been unfaithful to him or because he has lost someone dear to him; we can see that he suffers—and suffers because of the accident that provoked his breakdown. But this understanding cannot fully account for his depression, his disgust with life, his general inertia, etc.—in fact, for the general pathological picture that his depression presents. 'Much as we may understand the original experience, the significance of the psychological trauma and the content of the reactive state, their particular transposition into the realm of the pathological remains psychologically incomprehensible to us.'[23]

We can only understand feelings we can ourselves experience; one has to be mad to understand madness. It is a different world from our own and it is difficult for us to find a way of entering it. Since we cannot understand madness, we tend to reconstruct it according to the models of normal psychology. We must therefore find an application for the case study outside the field of *verstehen*.

We believe that it is best applied in the way that 'life histories' are used in general sociology and in anthropology.[24] Case histories can either suggest hypotheses to the sociologist, or support them, or at least illustrate them with well-chosen examples. They can suggest hypotheses in the following way: Psychoanalysis implies, for example, that the sociologist should give a great deal of importance to early experience in the aetiology of mental disturbance. Freud and his successors have provided us with numerous detailed case analyses showing the influence of early experience. This suggests a research hypothesis that the sociologist may accept, providing, of course, that it can be statistically tested. It also raises problems, since statistical analysis requires that variables be quantifiable. For example, let us consider child-rearing practices without taking into account the total parent-child relationship. Sewell studied the effects of weaning and toilet-training on 162 American farm children; he observed that breast-fed children who were weaned gradually did not differ from those weaned abruptly. Toilet-training, on the other hand, seemed to have an effect, depending on whether it was undertaken early or late, but the children who were trained by being punished did not differ from those who were not punished. This does not mean, of course, that the Freudian hypothesis must be rejected, but we do have a partial answer which is objectively verified: it is not the actual practice which is important, but the overall atmosphere in which these childhood experiences occur[25]— in other words, the father-mother-child relationship.

We come closer to this relationship in our second example. Basing himself on clinical observations, Arieti suggested that paranoid forms of schizophrenia develop in children whose mothers are not critical of their actions, but of their bad thoughts, whereas catatonic forms develop in children who cannot act by themselves because their parents take all their decisions for them. Thus we find at the origin of two pathological types two different kinds of parental behaviour: rejection and over-protection.[26] This type of hypothesis suggested by case studies can only be accepted by the sociologist if he can submit it, at least indirectly, to statistical testing. Table 1, taken from Sanua's book, gives the distribution of rejection and over-protection in two groups of families, Jewish and Protestant.

We may therefore conclude that case studies can suggest hypotheses. These hypotheses cannot all be tested directly or indirectly, but they are obviously only part of the sociological study of mental disorder if they have subsequently been given sociological treatment.

In the second place, case histories can be useful either as illustrations or concrete examples to clarify certain questions, or as instruments for the testing of hypotheses. We shall give one example which will be dealt with at greater length in another chapter. According to Faris and Dunham, there is a statistically significant link between schizophrenia and residence in urban areas of social disorganization, which points to isolation as a causative factor in schizophrenia. But the figures only show the tendency for schizophrenics to reside in certain neighbourhoods; they do not say anything about the causes of the illness. Only life histories can take us from correlations to explanations. What the life histories of these psychotics do show is that in most cases the childhood of the patients was normal and free of schizophrenic symptoms; illness developed later in the isolation of socially disorganized neighbourhoods.[27]

A fruitful dialogue is thus established between the sociologist and the psychiatrist, and their methods, although apparently contradictory, since one is oriented towards the general and the other towards the particular, prove to be complementary. Is a similar dialogue possible between the anthropologist and the sociologist? We will deal with this question much more briefly. We have already noted that in ethnopsychiatry the basic method is the comparative one (which can take several forms, but which most

Table 1   Parental rejection and over-protection among Jewish and Protestant schizophrenics

	Paranoid Jews	Catatonic Jews	Paranoid Protestants	Catatonic Protestants
Paternal rejection	10	2	10	11
Maternal rejection	7	7	10	0
Rejection by both parents	17	7	15	0
Paternal rejection and maternal over-protection	12	2	6	4
Paternal over-protection	2	2	2	4
Maternal over-protection	27	43	16	35
Both parents over-protective	2	3	2	4
Other	23	35	39	37

An analysis of the above figures will show some differences between the Jewish and Protestant schizophrenics as well as differences between the paranoids and catatonics. More parental rejection was found among families of Protestant schizophrenics and, conversely, more over-protection was found among the Jewish families. A comparison of the incidence of rejection among families with paranoid schizophrenics as against families with catatonic schizophrenics indicates that the frequency is two or three times higher among the former group.[28]

often today consists of cross-cultural studies). The sociology of mental disorder, on the other hand, deals with a single cultural area. More than his particular technique of investigation, it is the anthropologist's approach to his material that has the most to offer.[29]

The most striking thing to the anthropologist is 'otherness'. There is, of course, a limit to this otherness, since no comparisons are possible without some basic identity or equivalence of meaning. But what he is aware of first and foremost is the diversity of symptomatologies from culture to culture. His basic rule is therefore to overcome his ethnocentric attitudes and not assess neurosis and psychosis in other cultures according to the categories created by Western psychiatry. In a previous book we pointed out the error of equating the child, the psychotic and primitive man, who until recently were still apt to be treated as identical.[30] It is none the less true that all three in different ways present the same problem of 'otherness' in an acute form. The advice of the ethnopsychiatrist who tries to be aware of the idiosyncrasies of different civilizations can be profitable to the psychiatrist. It can help him to overcome what Sullivan called his 'cultural handicap', the fact that he moves in a different world from his patient.[31] But it is the attitude rather than the technique which is valuable and more so for social psychiatry than for the sociology of mental disorder. The latter field will probably make more use of the results of ethnopsychiatry than of its methods. The present century is marked by a tremendous mixing of people and civilizations. Individuals or families migrate, either temporarily or permanently, of their own free will or under pressure. Migrants take with them and preserve for a long time their ways of feeling and thinking, their 'basic personalities' which are a product of their formative years and of all the subtle influences of their cultural *milieu*. They remain attached to their old values. The sociologist who aims to study migrants is obliged to turn his attention first of all to this phenomenon of internalized culture if he is to understand the particular modes of response of migrants to their new environment. Thus when Raveau studies neurosis among African immigrants in Paris, it is difficult to decide whether he does so as an ethnopsychiatrist or as a sociologist.

4 Interdisciplinary research

Everything points to the conclusion that a close working relationship is necessary between the psychiatrist, the sociologist and, in some research at least, the anthropologist. This means that in a field as complex as the one we are about to tackle, psychiatrist and sociologist must not remain isolated, but must work as a team. Interdisciplinary research has its own particular rules; since they are not always recognized by methodologists of the social sciences, we must try as far as we can to remedy this regrettable failure.

It is, of course, possible to imagine a psychiatric interested in sociology who applies the findings of sociology to his own case analyses or who tries to develop a psychiatrist sociology. Similarly, one can imagine a sociologist interested in psychiatry who develops his theories by studying mental hospital files or by administering special questionnaires to certain categories of patients. We need only refer back to our first chapter to see that this is how both the sociology of mental illness and social psychiatry were born. Nevertheless, specialization is increasing every day, and it is impossible to know everything. The psychiatrist who tries his hand at sociology runs the risk of committing serious errors in all good faith, just as the sociologist who is interested in psychiatry finds himself in a field where his training is inadequate; even if he is trained, he is unlikely to have had the long practical experience of the professional psychiatrist. It is therefore essential for each specialist to keep the other in order. This mutual process of control raises ethical and methodological problems which are rather difficult to overcome.

The Americans are especially sensitive to the ethical problems. They distinguish two types of interdisciplinary research: the 'autocratic' and the 'democratic', according to whether there is a research leader or different specialists on an equal footing. One often finds in American sociological journals complaints by sociologists against the authoritarianism of medical men, who seem to want to direct co-operative research at all costs. Naturally, the democratic ideal should remain the ethical norm for interdisciplinary study (the methodological norm is another question). But as this research is carried out by human beings, their particular enthusiasms, even if ethically pure (that is, arising not from a desire to dominate, but from a belief in the value of the field they have chosen), create tensions and provoke conflicts of authority. In addition to this first difficulty there is the problem of particular cliques in sociology and psychiatry, and the conflict between different schools, which is particularly bitter in some countries. The sociologist and the psychiatrist are so closely identified with their theories, often the fruit of long and painstaking research, that they find it extremely difficult to accept a point of view different from their own. Their particular truth becomes *the* truth. Some are even afraid of surrendering what has become a part, and often the best part, of their personality to interdisciplinary discussion. If they do agree to do so, it is often with the idea that their point of view will triumph over other people's. These are, of course, commonplace remarks; nevertheless, interdisciplinary research is a necessity of our time, and it will probably become more so in the future—hence this appeal for self-denial.

The methodology of interdisciplinary research is governed by the fact that joint conclusions must be reached. On a practical level, this means that a decision must be taken by the group. We are interested in the rules governing this decision. First of all, there is the method used by Leighton and his collaborators in America and more recently in Nigeria. It consists in giving each member of the research team maximum autonomy—freedom to work in his own field with his own methods. A director reads the reports, compares them, and extracts a certain number of hypotheses and conclusions. Naturally, informal discussions take place, so that there is some link between the investigators, but democracy in discussions does not rule out the fact that there is a research 'leader'. Nevertheless, the autonomy of the various branches is maintained until the end, and the resulting book, where each chapter is the work of one or two authors, is a good expression of a co-existence which tends strongly towards unity.[32] The Community Survey Operation, which we mentioned before, was aimed at the detection in a very large community of mental disturbance that was not treated in hospital. Psychologists were given the task of administering the American Army Neuropsychiatric Questionnaire, the Minnesota Multiphasic Inventory, etc., but the material collected was then examined by psychiatrists, who drew conclusions from it. The work of Kardiner is the result of a collaboration between himself, a psychoanalyst, and an anthropologist, Linton: the anthropologist mainly collected the material to be analysed and in the end the psychoanalyst had the crucial role.[33] This method of interdisciplinary research undoubtedly has advantages, in that it makes decisions quicker and easier. It does not preclude democracy in work-relationships—in fact, it is conducive to it in that it gives each group of workers as much autonomy as possible in their particular field. Nevertheless, this is the sort of research we would call 'stratified'; it implies super-imposed levels, with psychiatry at the top.

A second method very much in use today in the U.S.A. presents the results of interdisciplinary research in an 'integrated' form. We can assume that the psychiatrist will play the principal role in locating patients and classifying them into operational psychiatric categories, while the sociologist will mainly contribute his statistical knowledge. But in reading the articles and books produced in this way we are not aware of this likely division of labour. The results are deliberately presented in a unified form. A good example is the study of mental illness and social class in the U.S.A. by Redlich, a psychiatrist, and Hollingshead, a sociologist.[34] One cannot help wondering, though, whether the modesty of the conclusions reached is not due to a certain fear of stepping over the bounds of pleasant co-operation and coming into conflict. In general the studies give correlations between age, sex, economic status, educational level, religion or the degree of social cohesiveness of a group and the frequency of a particular form of mental disorder. But they do not tell us why and often not even how these correlations come about. It may well be that for many sociologists the establishment of facts is sufficient in itself, but these facts are surely indicators—as Durkheim shows in *Suicide*—of factors other than individual ones—namely, social factors. Hence the suggestion that integrated interdisciplinary research tends to stop at a certain level so as to avoid the disruption of egalitarian co-operation and the risk of awakening a conflict of opinion.

The aims of interdisciplinary research are no different from those of individual research: the substitution of a constructed object for a given object, or what used to be known as the transformation of common-sense knowledge into scientific knowledge. Bachelard lays down the conditions for the construction of an object either by an individual scientist or by a team of people who are nevertheless members of the same specialized field, when he discusses the mental mechanisms and rationalist techniques needed to attain precision: 'for the construction of a precise object we need precise thinking. Precise thinking is thinking which is open to debate on its precision. If we go to the root of the divergent tendencies, it is obvious that precision is an instance of the I-Thou relationship.'[35]

The scientist must be open to the supervision of others. In interdisciplinary research these other people, the supervisors, belong to other branches of learning, which complicates the rules of 'applied rationalism'. Bachelard's dialectic has then to be reversed. Bachelard demonstrated that the *cogito* of the scientist is only valid when it becomes a *cogitamus*, that of the 'union of workers seeking proof'. But here we have a *cogitamus* which must be transformed into a *cogito*. The aim is to introduce mutual suspicion among those working on the construction of an object, to 'energize' the process of approbation by going from one proof to another proof in a different field: the psychiatrist challenges the sociologist, who takes up the challenge; the psychiatrist in turn casts doubt upon the objectivity of the sociologist's construction, etc. As each feeling of mistrust is overcome, as each proof calls for a new proof, either biological, chemical, medical, psychological or sociological, bit by bit a scientific object is constructed whose logical coherence is only the expression, or the result, of the sociological agreement of the Is and Thous. The dialogue gives birth to a unified object, and finally dies out because this 'oneness' is a joint achievement. This seems to be the direction in which the new generation of research workers are moving.[36]

The questions arising, then, are no longer the ones we mentioned at first. Is there a predominant point of view, and whose is it? Who is to have the last word and conclude the debate? Should the team preferably be led by a psychiatrist or by a sociologist? The various techniques have finally been drawn together in a plethora of proofs and counter-proofs and the debate between different disciplines has become a 'union of workers seeking proof'. But it is important to understand the following idea: so long as the object of study remains external to the scientist, no science can be anything more than a light thrown on the object, and there is no way at all of deciding which 'competitor's' light is the truest. The assessment would have to be made on a higher plane and there is no such thing as a 'super-science'. Therefore, as Bachelard suggests, the external object must be transformed and replaced by a scientific 'construction', all sciences being in the end systems of rules of construction. Interdisciplinary work then becomes possible, which is not to say that it is easy. A system must now be constructed with several avenues of approach. Whereas in the study that only intends to be empirical the insoluble problem is the absence of a super-science to solve any arguments that arise as to who is finally right, here, on the contrary, we know when the work is finished. The coherence of the constructed object, which is both a logical and sociological coherence, is evidence of the completion—only temporary, of course—of the interdisciplinary study. There is no need for recourse to some *deus ex machina*—in this case the research director.

5   The experimental method

Ever since the beginnings of sociology this has been an important issue for sociologists who wish to model the human sciences on the natural sciences. From Comte to Durkheim the comparative method tended to be regarded as a substitute for the experimental method. Variables in this case are obviously not manipulated as in physics or chemistry, the changes observed being 'natural', but subsequent observation can show that these changes are not due to chance, but occur in relation to the transformation of one or other element of the whole. This method is known today as *ex post facto* experimentation. However, at the time of the Russian Revolution Mauss welcomed the Soviet's deliberate manipulation of social factors to achieve definite ends, and he came to the interesting conclusion that politics is a sort of sociological experiment. From then on, in step with the development of idealistic planning, another type of experimental research began to appear: it equates planning with applied sociology (the critical examination of the deliberate manipulation of the elements of a social structure by social reformers). In both these types of experiment, however, in spite of refinements in method, one is never sure of controlling all the variables: the hidden factors in a society are more important than what is manifest.

Hence the growing importance of the small-group study. We referred to this in the previous chapter in connection with Moreno and the French school of sociometry. It consists in reproducing experimentally the simplest possible situations for the testing of particular working hypotheses. For example, two small groups can be set up, one with a democratic régime and the other with an authoritarian régime, to see whether one is more efficient than the other in solving a particular problem. The difficulties encountered by this method are obvious: Is it possible to generalize without the risk of committing errors from an artificially constituted group to a 'natural' group, even a small one, such as the family or the neighbourhood? What right has one to extrapolate from the results of 'micro-sociology', as the Americans call it, to the macrosociological field? If democracy in small groups proves conducive to better problem-solving, does this necessarily infer the superiority of the democratic over the authoritarian system on a national scale?

Relevant though these criticisms are to small-group sociology in general, they fortunately do not apply, or at least apply less, when we switch from normal groups to psychologically disturbed groups. This is because we are dealing with normally artificial groups; in other words, artificiality in the mental hospital is, scientifically speaking, the rule. The next reason is that the function of the hospital is to cure the patient, and all processes of cure involve a manipulation of body or mind; therefore manipulation, which is arbitrary in classical small-group sociology, is seen by the scientist to be the rule within the hospital walls. Finally, this manipulation has more and more over the last few years taken the form of group therapy—in other words, therapeutic necessity has forced psychiatrists to organize 'small groups'. With abnormal as opposed to normal subjects we have all the elements of a valid small-group sociology that for the most part evades the criticisms mentioned earlier, on condition, of course, that one does not generalize to normal people the results of experiments made with groups of mental patients. We shall give some examples of this type of experiment to assess its potential value.

The chairs occupied by patients can be placed in a semicircle, in a circle round a table or in a row, and each patient can be assigned to a particular place. But the best way is not to arrange the chairs before the session and to ask patients to sit wherever they like. One then notices that those in need of security sit next to the therapist, while those whose behaviour is passive and who have difficulties in social participation tend to sit as far as possible from the therapist—for example, at the extremities of the semicircle.

Particularly anxious individuals also sit at the extremities, as a feeling of being closed in only intensifies their anxiety. They choose a seat from which they can leave the group as easily as possible. Besides this choice of seats resulting from personal disturbances, there are other types of choice caused by normal sociability. For example, patients who are in the habit of meeting outside the sessions sit next to each other and form what amounts to subgroups within the group. Experiments can be carried out by varying these two factors which affect the patients' location and by observing the results. First of all, the personality factor can be varied. Thus a hysterical woman who has difficulties in social interaction, especially with men, and who under analysis has shown that her aggressive attitude towards her father is expressed by a constant wish to occupy a superior position, always sits opposite the therapist. The therapist only needs to point out the Oedipal origin of her disturbance for her first of all to stop coming to the group, then to sit at the edge of the semicircle, and finally to occupy any chair that happens to be free. Secondly, one can vary the sociological factor by introducing social 'isolates', generally newcomers, into subgroups of friends. We cannot describe this type of experiment in detail. However, the conclusion that emerges is that the social space of mentally-ill people is structured like ours, but follows different rules. The patient's distance from the centre, represented in this case by the therapist, is determined by his ego defence mechanisms, while sociologically normal elements introduced into the group will tend to conform to other structural rules determined by affective ties and will therefore tend to split the therapeutic group into several subgroups.[37]

It has often been debated whether the therapeutic group should be homogeneous or heterogeneous. A more interesting question is what happens when an outsider is introduced into a homogeneous group. The 'stranger' is always considered 'strange' and is therefore ambiguous to the existing group: he often becomes the enemy. This phenomenon was studied by Simmel (*Sociologie*). We shall therefore describe a second type of experiment: the introduction into a group of a deviant in relation to the norms of the group. We do not mean, of course, a sociological deviant—for example, a man in a group of women (he might well take an interest in one of the women and thus provoke a crisis in the group detrimental to recovery, which is after all the therapist's end), nor, for example, a Negro in a group of white Americans (the white people would no longer express themselves freely in case the Negro should feel the victim of general hostility and seek revenge: where this experiment has been tried, this fear is revealed in the dreams of the white patients). We mean, on the contrary, a pathological deviant, a patient belonging to a different nosological category from that of the group. Here again the therapist anxious to effect a cure has to limit the extent of his experiments; he would not, for example, introduce an epileptic, as he might have an attack during the session. The introduction of what we termed 'sociological deviants' does not in fact create different problems from those which can be observed in everyday life: an American is put in quarantine by a group of English people; a group wants to initiate a newly arrived young man to sex, etc. But when a schizophrenic is placed in a non-schizophrenic group he will begin to make efforts to express himself and communicate with the others; he will feel encouraged to participate actively. When a heterosexual is introduced into a group of homosexuals, on the one hand the homosexuals are able to understand better the latent conflicts that produced the heterosexual's neurosis, and are able to reveal them to him, and on the other hand the heterosexual tends to become a 'propagandist' and to convert the other members of the group. The conclusion emerging from these experiments is that the acceptance of the deviant by the group reassures him about his problems, lessens and finally eliminates his anxiety and his reaction of fear.[38] In addition, the experiments suggest that the therapist is a 'deviant', too, sometimes sociologically (for example, if he belongs to a religious or ethnic minority) but also pathologically speaking (in that he belongs to a world that is considered normal). Consequently, the group-therapy process can tell us, in the particular case of the introduction of outsiders into small groups, about the possible ways of overcoming what we called earlier the cultural handicap of the psychiatrist.

Up to now we have only mentioned experiments conducted 'just to see'. Given the present primitive state of research, it is difficult to go further than this in the experimental field. However, there is an inevitable trend towards controlled experiments which are infinitely more fruitful for the development of science. Thus we have an experiment such as the one made by Courchet and Maucorps, who discovered, or, rather, rediscovered, a psychiatric entity which they named 'lightning psychosis' (*psychose éclair*), a psychosis that disappears as suddenly as it appears. According to them, it is found mainly in particular groups, such as farm labourers working on large estates and unskilled workers lost in the anonymity of city life, both groups being deprived of any link with the community. This led them to the hypothesis that, besides alienation and exploitation, the mere fact of a 'social vacuum' is sufficient to produce disturbance. To test this hypothesis they developed a group-therapy technique which they called *apétotherapie*. This consisted in fighting the apathy of the patients by awakening their sense of protest. The hypothesis is verified by a thorough quantitative analysis.[39]

As the authors emphasize in their conclusions, this method ought really to be compared with occupational and play-therapy with similar patients, to check whether the active element in the thera-peutic process is the content of the task (the patients' assertion of their rights) or merely the fact that there is a common task to be performed which can only be done by an organized group.

Thus as research grows from day to day, new methods of investi-gation appear and old ones are continually being perfected. We have at our disposal more and more precise means for the develop-ment of a sociology of mental disorder. What results have these new methods produced?

III Prolegomena to a sociology of mental disorder

Before we deal with the empirical studies and their results, a few preliminary questions must be answered. In our previous historical and methodological discussion we repeatedly encountered such concepts as 'normal' and 'pathological', the definition of which we shelved for the time being, or else very general problems whose solution we left until later—for example, whether or not mental illness can have social causes. Our historical review and the methods we have described imply that social factors do in fact operate at both psychological and physical levels. All the empirical studies we shall review in the following chapters postulate the existence of social factors in mental illness and endeavour to discover them. Are these assumptions based on an illusion? We can no longer put off the examination of this question. However, even if we should discover in the end that the 'biologists' are right and the 'sociologists' are wrong, would not a sociology of mental disorder still have a right to exist, given that it were founded on different principles? Where would we look for these principles?

The present chapter will be devoted to the prolegomena to the development of a sociological theory of mental pathology. First let us define what we mean by 'normal' and 'pathological'.

1 What is a pathological case?

Normal means that which conforms to the norm. But since each civilization has its own system of norms, cannot what is normal in one civilization be considered pathological in another, or vice versa? We can see the importance of this question in ethnopsychiatry. If we use the definition of the sociology of mental illness that we constructed in the Introduction of this book, we could to a certain extent ignore the problem, since both patient and psychiatrist belong to the same civilization and therefore to the same system of norms. Public opinion is in agreement on the criteria distinguishing the 'sane' from the 'insane'. However, it is not entirely possible to ignore the arguments between anthropologists and psychiatrists on the relativity of normality and pathology, as ideas have gradually emerged from these arguments that have a bearing, not only on ethnopsychiatry, but on sociology as well.

The debate started with the famous and often-quoted article by Ruth Benedict, 'Anthropology and the Abnormal'.[1] She refers to a certain number of facts gathered by anthropologists, such as the normality of the trance in shamanistic societies, of homosexuality in 'berdache' societies, the paranoid character of Melanesian cultures (Dobu) and the encouragement of megalomania by the Kwakiutl. She concludes that what are considered in the West to be pathological states are in fact regarded as quite normal in societies other than our own. This is because the concept of 'normality' is a variation on the concept of 'goodness': a normal action is a good action, sanctioned by the community and corresponding to the group ideal. Kwakiutl culture is based on the custom of the *potlatch*, or competition for prestige: we may consider the paranoid personality to be pathological, but the Kwakiutl see it, on the contrary, as highly desirable, since it underlies their traditions of jousting, challenges and competitions of gifts. What is more, a child's whole education is aimed at cultivating and developing the germ of paranoia; the child who is too passive, gentle or submissive will be considered 'abnormal'. In the same way suspiciousness taking the form of delusions of persecution is interpreted in our culture as mental disturbance; but to the Dobuans suspicions are never considered to have imaginary causes: they are part of a 'magical' culture where the unpredictable attacks of the witchdoctor are to be feared at all times. Naturally, the individual who is predisposed to suspiciousness is fully adapted to the traditional values, and it is the aim of the culture to force those who are not similarly inclined into the common pattern.

Ruth Benedict's warning against the ethnocentrism of psychiatrists has been very useful. It was too often taken for granted that our psychiatric frames of reference were universal and valid for all times and places. She asks us not to judge other cultures according to our own value systems or our ideal models of behaviour, as though all men could be equated with Western man. And yet one can detect a trace of ethnocentrism in Ruth Benedict's attitude, which becomes apparent in her endless comparisons of primitive societies with our own. After all, she does base the relativity of normality and pathology on the categories discovered and classified by Western psychiatry (mystical hysteria, paranoia, etc.). When the behaviour patterns that seem to us pathological are in fact dictated by the norms of the society, we should no longer speak of the relativity of abnormality, since we are no longer in the realm of pathology, but are dealing with normal cultural processes. To correct this tendency, Foley suggested a statistical criterion of abnormality.[2] He probably took Ruth Benedict as a starting-point, but he succeeded better than she did in eliminating his last traces of ethnocentrism. Abnormal behaviour, according to Foley, is behaviour 'deviating' from the norm—that is from the central tendency of the population, from the general behaviour of the group. Normal behaviour is the behaviour prevalent at a given moment; it is the most common, the one showing the highest rate of occurrence. Foley's criterion certainly has a merit which has not been sufficiently emphasized: it represents an effort to remove the problem of pathology from the subjectivity of value-judgments so as to give it a scientific basis. Not that it eliminates values, but values are considered as collective 'facts' both observable and quantifiable, and not as 'value-judgments'. A similar attempt to produce an objective definition of pathology is found in Durkheim's *Rules of Scientific Method*, except that Durkheim rejected the identification of normal with average. Maries Jahoda points out that whereas Foley's criterion can be applied in anthropological studies of small societies, it is no longer valid in sociology—that is, for societies like our own, where there is on the whole less uniformity and where one must take into account not only the mean of the behaviour curve, but also its extremities.[3] Wegrocki, on the other hand, notes that statistics imply a relative scale (one is more or less paranoid); they do not draw a line between normal and pathological. There are, of course, certain abnormalities that can be graded on a scale, but others cannot be measured in this way, as they belong to a different substratum. In fact, statistics can only be used for observable behaviour, in which case they can show deviations from the norm. However, a type of behaviour cannot be called pathological just because it deviates from the general behaviour of the group; the important factor is the 'cause' of the phenomenon. For example, the reason why the hallucinations of the Plains Indians are not abnormal is not that they are a usual phenomenon, a norm imposed by the culture, but that the hallucinations are not produced by an inner conflict, as with schizophrenics in our culture. In a sentence that admirably sums up his thinking, Wegrocki concludes: 'The "abnormal" behaviour of the Indian is analogous to the behaviour of the psychotic but not homologous.'[4]

This discussion leads us from 'culturalism' back to Western psychiatry with its categories, regarded as universally valid, from which Ruth Benedict wanted us to escape. In the end it is the psychiatrist and the psychiatrist alone who is capable of defining the criteria that distinguish pathological from normal behaviour. For Wegrocki the criteria are a reaction of escape when faced with inner conflict, plus constitutional elements or lesions. For Hsu, the mentally-ill person is an individual pursued by his own past, i.e. his infantile experience, to the extent of not being able to adapt to his present situation;[5] the normal person represses his past to adjust to the present. The view that the psychiatrist alone is capable of defining the pathological case is generally the view of French psychiatrists. They do accept that some psychotic syndromes can take on a different aspect in different cultures, that instinctual behaviour can follow different patterns according to the life-style of the ethnic group, but the 'primary' disturbance behind the superficial trappings is something constant, and is determined by biological dysfunctions.[6] Whereas cultural factors can vary, the characteristic of biological factors is that they obey universal and fixed rules. American psychiatry is more reticent, even when it criticizes Benedict or Foley. At times it accepts eclectically all three criteria, the cultural, the statistical and the clinical, but it applies them to different spheres of abnormality. Morgan, for example, maintains that the first criterion is valid for the psychoneuroses, the second for sexual abnormalities or disturbances that are barely pathological, and the third for functional psychoses.[7] At other times it superimposes the psychiatric criterion and the cultural one. Kluckhohn points out that among 'deviants' one always finds the mentally ill: 'All cultures *must* regard as abnormal individuals whose behaviour fails grossly to be predictable in accord with cultural norms, or (and here is the important addition) who are permanently inaccessible to communication, or who consistently lack a certain minimum of control over their impulse life.'[8]

Or else we have Linton's distinction between absolute abnormality, which has a constitutional basis and is found in all societies, and relative abnormality, which measures the degree to which certain personality configurations are at variance with the basic culturally determined personality.[9] Anthropological research confirms this point of view. It seems, indeed, that all societies differentiate between several types of abnormality, one of which actually corresponds to what our psychiatrists would call mental disorder. To give only one example, the Australian Aborigines differentiate between the super-normal 'strong-men' (Margidjbus), who are gifted with supernatural powers; the 'infra-normal' (Bengwar) men, who are not outsiders, but who do not behave like everyone else (which is applying the cultural criterion) and, finally, the 'victims of sorcery', who have been robbed of their spirits and are the actual equivalent of our madmen (psychiatric criterion).[10] What remains of the argument for cultural relativism? (1) The probable fact—even though it is not proven statistically—of the unequal distribution of various types of mental disorder according to race and civilization. Buddhism, for example, is considered to protect the schizoid personality through its ascetic practices and escape from reality, thus preventing the development of full-blown schizophrenia. There is perhaps two to three times less schizophrenia in India than in America. (2) The diversity of forms that a disorder can take from culture to culture; in other words, the relativity of symptoms (Arctic hysteria, Amok seizure, *witigo* among the Canadian Indians, Malaysian *koro*, etc.). (3) The fact that certain types of individual can be tolerated in one culture and not in another, and that the culture can even provide institutionalized models enabling these individuals to be integrated into society.[11]

We have just summarized, as briefly as possible, a debate that has involved anthropologists and psychiatrists for the past twenty or twenty-five years. However, we have left aside a number of questions on the fringe of the debate which we must now treat more fully. Although, as we have seen, the general debate is mainly concerned with ethnopsychiatry, a certain number of other topics arise in connection with it which we shall now examine because of their particular relevance to the subject of this book, the sociology of mental disorder.

The reader will recall the gist of the relativist argument as we defined it according to Ruth Benedict: normal is that which conforms to the norm and pathological is that which deviates from it. Hence the question asked by anthropologists and psychiatrists alike: Can deviance be equated with pathological abnormality? Parsons defines deviance as a reluctance or an inability of the ego to internalize certain rules or even to make its behaviour conform to social norms. He lists four possible personality types: the overconformist, the rebel, the ritualist and the escapist. Although neurotics may be more likely than others to be ritualists or escapists, the point is that deviance is a sociological and not a psychiatric phenomenon. When French sociologists speak of 'marginality', which is the approximate equivalent of the Anglo-Saxon term 'deviance', they classify as marginal those immigrants who are not yet settled, criminals, prostitutes and tramps, along with the mentally ill. Of course, the tramp may be feeble-minded and the criminal paranoid, just as the immigrant may go through a neurotic crisis at some point in his life, but social marginality must not be confused with psychiatric abnormality. Ruth Benedict's error would seem to be that she combined two naturally heterogeneous facts, cultural normality and mental health, no doubt because they are often linked. She generalized the relativity of the former (each culture having its own type of deviant) to the latter type of normality, which is individually and not culturally based.[12] Devereux has perhaps succeeded best in clarifying this confused situation.[13] He points out in the first place that social adjustment is not, from the psychiatric point of view, a sign of mental health: conformism can take pathological forms, in particular sado-masochism. Secondly, he emphasizes that maladjustment is more a consequence than a cause of mental disorder, and that it is therefore more a source of problems to the psychiatrist than a useful criterion. He reveals the hidden postulate of cultural relativism, which is that only individuals can be ill and that society is always normal. This would seem to be a new version of the old adage, *Vox populi, vox Dei.* We shall return later on in this chapter to the question of sick societies; it is obvious that if societies can be sick, the individual internalizing the norms of the collectivity is internalizing sick norms. Rebellion in this case, and not adjustment, is the true sign of health. In contradiction to Ruth Benedict and her followers, he shows that the *shaman* is in fact, psychiatrically speaking, neurotic, even if he is adapted to a social function. This is because it is necessary to differentiate between the ethnic or cultural unconscious, which includes all that is repressed by the society, and the individual unconscious. The neurotic conflicts of the *shaman* belong to the ethnic unconscious and not to the idiosyncratic part of his personality. This is why he can control his impulses and ritualize his conflicts according to the conventions of his social group. But besides the cultural unconscious which allows for the integration of anti-social behaviour into society, another deeper unconscious comes into play, the unconscious of psychotics and neurotics who have experienced culturally atypical traumas. In this case the group is unable to provide traditional defence mechanisms. Thus we can see that the question of the relationship between social adjustment (for the *shaman* this is in fact an adjustment to a relatively marginal sector of society) and mental disorder is much more complicated than cultural relativism maintains: adjustment is not the criterion of health.

But one can also understand what led Ruth Benedict to her relativist conception of mental illness: although psychiatrists were opposed to it, they were the ones who suggested it to her in the first place. Given a definition of pathology as a failure to adjust to the physical and social environment, and given that the social environment varies from one group to another, adjustment can only be as relative and unstable as the environment. We need therefore to go beyond this psychiatric definition. This was well understood by Goldstein, for example, who defined normal as 'normative' and not as an adjustment to norms.[14] A sick organism can be adapted to a restricted environment. Aphasic patients can adjust to a concrete level of behaviour by limiting the scope of their communication; neurotics can likewise find a niche sheltered from serious difficulties where they can continue to live 'normally'. The healthy individual, on the contrary, is the one who can strike back at a complex and changing world and devise new norms of behaviour at a moment's notice; his adjustment to the environment is less important than his ability to modify it. Canguilhem reached similar conclusions.[15] It is possible, he maintains, to give an objective description of structures and behaviour, but in judging whether they should be called 'pathological' one can rely on no objective criterion. 'Normal' and 'pathological' are concepts that lead us into the realm of values. It is only with reference to the dynamic polarity of life that we can apply the term 'normal' to certain personalities or certain functions. Life is not only submission to the environment, but also the setting up of one's own environment, a perpetual act of renewal and creativity. From this point of view, illness is indeed a lifestyle, but an inferior one, in the sense that it does not tolerate any irregularities in the conditions of life; it is conservative and tied to the environment. A person is healthy to the extent that he remains normative in relation to the fluctuations of the environment, is able to evolve different models of behaviour, change his mode of response, and transform his life-circumstances. The sick man is only cured when he can set himself new norms. To a certain degree we find the same idea in Marie Jahoda's work, when she tries to define the criteria of mental health and lists the following three: adjustment to the environment, unity of personality, correct perception of reality. Each of these criteria, she says, can be criticized when taken separately. The correct perception of reality (including one's own psychological reality) is difficult to attain; many people never achieve it and yet are considered normal. Unity of personality also exists in catatonic states, and the criterion is only valid if it means unity in richness, not in poverty of the self. As for adjustment to the environment (and this is where we discover that she is related to Goldstein and Canguilhem) it is not sufficient as a criterion, for the sane person is one who can achieve independence from the pressures and influences of the situation in which he finds himself, who chooses, in fact, or who creates.[16]

At this point we cannot help feeling a little worried. Contemporary thinkers seem to have given the best definitions of 'normal' and 'pathological'. Were they not in fact using their common sense? Surely the psychiatric criterion ends up by being similar to the popular distinction between 'mad' and 'sane'. Ruth Benedict has not yet been exorcised. Although, as we said before, her theory is an ethnopsychiatric one, this is the reason we could not leave her out of our sociology of mental illness. We shall have occasion to return at the end of this book to the distinction the community makes between madness and sanity: the insane person is one who of his own accord goes to a psychiatrist for treatment, or the person whose confinement is requested either by his relatives or by the police. The dividing line between the two realms varies, as we shall see, from group to group within the same society. Thus it is never entirely possible to escape from relativity. The function of the psychiatrist is to search for the 'causes', to report on the 'whys' of the illness, but society decides who his patients will be. There is a subtle play of influences between the doctor and the public. The doctor, through the mass media or other agencies, tends to enlarge the field of mental illness, to make the public more aware of disturbances that are minor and have been until then attributed to 'oddness' or 'eccentricity'. On the other hand, he accepts the lay definition of mental illness, and his work is limited to refining or making more explicit this definition by introducing categories of 'insanity' (schizophrenia, manic-depressive psychosis, confusional states, etc.). But these categories never extend beyond the boundaries of insanity as defined by public opinion.

2   The importance of sociogenesis in the aetiology of mental disorder

Before we broach the question of the role of social factors—not in epidemiology, where there is more or less general agreement, but in aetiology, where controversy is often violent—it would seem useful to examine certain variables, such as sex, age or race, which are biological categories, to see whether they really behave like biological categories or more like social ones. We will not, of course, solve the problem, as these biological categories are universal and can tell us nothing about the pathological, but if they also act as social categories they will at least give us a first reliable indication of the possibility of sociogenesis in mental disturbance.

First of all, there is a difference in the rate of mental disorder between men and women; however, as the direction of the difference varies in different situations, it is not possible to state whether one sex is more vulnerable than the other. Thus in Brazil, until recently, there were more mentally sick men in the white population and more women among the Negroes. The only possible explanation, according to Nina Rodrigues, is that the white woman accepted the domination of her father and then of her husband, while the breadwinner bore all the responsibilities and had to tackle the everyday problems of existence.[17] On the other hand, after the abolition of slavery, Negro men were not able to integrate into the new class system, as they found that all the suitable jobs were already held by European immigrants. They became parasites on the Negro women who had found a way into the new social structure as maids, washerwomen or seamstresses, and who thus found themselves obliged to take on the family responsibilities. Therefore it is not sex as a biological category which is important, but the influence of sex as an organizational factor in society.

We come now to the age factor. The following average ages are given for first admissions to hospitals in the United States from 1929 to 1931:

Table 2 Age distribution of hospitalized patients in the U.S.A. (1929–31)

Psychiatric category	Age (in years)
Senile psychosis	74·5
Cerebral arteriosclerosis	66–63
Involutional melancholia and paranoia	53–50·3
General paresis and alcoholic psychosis	44·4–45·2
Dementia praecox	33·9
Manic-depressive psychosis	37
Psychoneurosis and neurosis	36·3
Psychopathic personality	35

This would seem to indicate that there are illnesses of youth (schizophrenia and psychosis linked with mental deficiency or epilepsy), of adulthood (manic-depressive psychosis, alcoholic psychosis and general paresis, followed by paranoia and involutional melancholia) and of old age (cerebral arteriosclerosis and senile psychosis).[18] But in relation to the illnesses of old age it is important not to confuse senility—a pathological phenomenon—with senescence, which is a normal stage in the life-cycle. The question is then whether senility is a consequence of ageing or rather an artificial product of a society where old people are rejected.[19] Répond has made the following comments on this subject:

> One cannot help wondering whether the old concept of senile dementia, thought to be the result of cerebral dysfunctions, should not be revised completely, and whether this pseudo-psychosis is not due to the patients' psycho-social condition, which rapidly deteriorates by placement in inadequately equipped and managed institutions as well as by confinement in psychiatric hospitals. The patients, often left to themselves, deprived of the necessary mental stimulation, cut off from all vital interests, are merely waiting for an end that one can hope will be rapid. We would even go so far as to suggest that the clinical picture of senile psychosis is an artifact most often due to a lack of care and preventive and rehabilitative treatment. After all, psychiatrists have believed almost up to this day in the more or less fatal evolution of insanity in most cases of schizophrenia. We now know that these discouraging syndromes were the result of a lack of appropriate psychological, social and medical care. They have disappeared in hospitals providing combined and active therapy. We can expect the same to happen with the classical syndromes of senile psychosis.

The psychological milestones marking the transition from one period of life to another which used to be considered particularly important in the causation of mental illness, such as the menopause, appear only to have an effect because of their social and symbolic significance rather than directly. The popular image of the menopause as the end of sexual life or as a crisis in interpersonal relations is the pathogenic influence.

Finally, we come to race in its accurate sense (not to be confused with ethnic group, which is synonymous with culture). This seems to be one of the biological factors which could account for the difference in the nature of mental disorder between Europeans, Asians and Africans. Aubin was one of the first to point out the contrast between the pattern of successive but discontinuous bouts of psychosis characteristic of Africans and the systematized and chronic pattern of Europeans. Carothers reminds us that the cerebral cortex and the epidermis derive from the same embryogenic element, the epiblast; it would therefore not be surprising if there were differences in the cerebral cortex between the two races, which would explain this differential pathology. Carothers draws our attention to the fact that cerebral convolutions, according to certain authors, are less pronounced in the African; the histological development of Africans is from seven to eight years behind that of Europeans. Without daring to admit it outright, he nevertheless implies that there is a biological basis for the lack of integration of the African personality. This lack of integration would explain the fact that their psychoses are relatively unstructured and take the form of brief attacks.[20] But this lack of ego integration could be due to many other factors, in particular tribal education, which replaces the authority of the father at the time of initiation by an external superego in the shape of the collective conscience. This would mean that with respect to psychiatric differences race is not so much a natural category as a cultural one.

This discussion of what has sometimes been called the 'biological dimension' of mental illness is not sufficient, without further study, to support the sociological hypothesis. It is merely an introduction to the idea of sociogenesis. Even if biological categories have an effect only through the intermediary of social factors, they still remain biological. The basic problem we shall now be concerned with is to know whether pathological states always derive in the final event from biological, constitutional or hereditary sources and how much importance, if any, we should give to social factors in the aetiology of mental disorder.

The history of psychiatry provides us with our first information.[21] In the earliest days people like Esquirol maintained that insanity had moral causes. Even Morel, in his theory of degeneration, does not discard the moral factor, but he already marks the beginning of a movement that seeks the final explanation in physical causes. This was followed by Magnan's concept of the hereditary taint, and then in the second half of the nineteenth century by the idea that the organism was responsible for mental disease. A search began for lesions affecting the brain and rigorously separate anatomical-clinical types were created, such as general paralysis of the insane, dementia praecox, manic-depressive psychosis, etc. This movement culminated in Kraepelin's systematic classification, which has long been the basis of psychiatric assessment. Naturally, there was some resistance. Lemoine, for example, in 1862, criticized the complacency of psychiatric explanations. Nothing is easier, he wrote, than to relate insanity always to an innate hidden predisposition, and to say that if the individual had had a different nature he would not have become insane. At the same time, with the influence of the German Romantics and their quest for laws governing symbolic thought, and with the growing interest in hypnotism and magnetism, another current was born that was to produce Freud's psychoanalysis. It placed the emphasis on the existence of mental disorder without organic links: the neuroses.

It seems that to understand this first period in the history of scientific psychiatry we must view it in the context of the various currents of nineteenth-century philosophical thought. In this particular period, to explain meant to reduce from the higher to the lower or, according to the Cartesian rule, from the complex to the simple. If the mind is an epiphenomenon of the body, then diseases of the mind can be reduced to diseases of the nervous system. The discovery of hereditary patterns only confirmed this belief among psychiatrists. The theory of constitutional types that can take both normal and pathological forms, the pathological being merely a caricature of the normal (as found in Dupré's writings in France or Kraepelin's classification of psychopathic entities), corresponds to a traditional philosophical conception going back as far as Aristotle. It is a theory of explanation by internal causality, according to which the behaviour of things is determined by their nature. The Galilean conception that things are determined by the conditions in which they happen, on which physics is based, had not yet reached the science of man. It was, of course, necessary to wait until it became accepted in all fields for a sociological conception of mental illness to appear—that is, until the twentieth century. This does not mean that the psychiatrists of the end of the nineteenth century did not draw on their own experience of life in evolving their theories, nor make wide use of clinical observations; but one should always be conscious of the philosophical or intellectual 'climate' in which doctrines develop and which necessarily influences them in a particular direction. The history of psychiatry does not therefore allow us to state that the concept of organogenesis is unfounded or at least exaggerated, but it does enable us to demystify it as a scientific theory. In our opinion it is more the expression of the philosophy of a given period than the product of objective research.

The twentieth century witnessed the reversal of the Aristotelian approach. We need not go over the history of the sociology of mental illness, to which we have already devoted a whole chapter. However, let us point out that the debate still continues between the supporters of sociogenesis and the supporters of organogenesis, with the difference that organogenetic theories have become much more plausible today.

To begin with, the theory of the hereditary nature of mental disease has been strengthened by the discovery of the laws of genetics. The importance of heredity is apparent in the concordance between twins of the transmission of schizophrenia. In identical twins the rate of concordance is 86·2 per cent and in fraternal twins 14·5 per cent. After having reviewed the entire literature on the genetic aspect of schizophrenia, Rosenthal concludes that the concordance of mental disorder (even if the illness does not lead to hospitalization) is higher in identical than in fraternal twins. There is, however, a margin between 86·2 per cent and 100 per cent which leaves a place for factors other than genetic. Jackson even concludes that the results of research on twins are not so convincing as they seem at first, for in no study have non-genetic factors been adequately controlled. The only thing we can conclude is that certain hosts are more receptive to mental disorder than others. To use Duchêne's words, illness, like combustion, requires both fuel and oxygen; the fact that both are necessary should not deter us from finding out their relative importance in modifying combustion. In other words, the genetic theory leaves room for sociogenesis.[22]

Above all, the laws of genetics necessarily operate within a social framework, and the effect of these laws depends on such factors as exogamy or endogamy, which are of a social nature. Consequently, culture has the final word in directing the course of heredity through marriage patterns (i.e. whether the choice of partner is enforced, selective or free); it can also determine mental hygiene and birth-control practices.[23] The genetic theory implies an *a priori* sociological standpoint; it does not invalidate it.

Babinski's theory, which distinguishes between lesional and functional disturbances, those due to an injury to the structure of the brain and those due to psychic causes, also allows for sociogenesis, in that it accepts that the psyche is inevitably moulded by society. It has been much discredited recently, since refined biochemical techniques have brought to light the action of diffuse factors as well as localized lesions, such as toxic, vascular and glandular factors affecting the entire nervous system. Hence the biochemical theories—of schizophrenia in particular—of Baruk in France, Buscaino in Italy or Heath in the U.S.A. I do not think they invalidate the idea of a sociology of mental illness. What better proof is there of this than the fact that Baruk has written a book on the ethical aspect of psychiatry and another on social psychiatry? Research in this field is still too recent to make a definite assessment possible; glandular disturbances can well be causally related to violent emotional shocks, which in turn can have a social origin. Some of the studies, in fact, were far too hastily made, as in the case of the urine analyses of schizophrenics and non-schizophrenics at the American Institute of Mental Health: it was found that the hospitalized schizophrenics drank coffee, and the substances in their urine thought to be characteristic of schizophrenia were simply due to the coffee. We must nevertheless bear the biochemical theory in mind, and we shall return to it in the last part of this book with a view to assessing its relevance in our field.[24]

In France the most severe criticism of the possibility of sociogenesis is that made by Henri Ey. It deserves more detailed examination. Ey is certainly not an adversary of social psychology, nor is he opposed to studying the social environment in order to understand the formation and development of personality. However, his opinion is that sociogenesis, although an established fact, can only explain normal man; the characteristic of pathological states is that sociogenesis ceases to apply.[25] It is impossible to understand disorganization, whether psychological or social, with reference to the forces of organization or of linkage between the individual and the outside world. This would be equivalent to explaining mental illness with reference to the laws governing health, which is a contradiction in terms. The realm of psychiatry is where psychogenesis ends (and all the more sociogenesis). If we do not accept that there is a difference in nature between the sane and the insane, as maintained, for example, by psychoanalysts who relate neurosis to man's basic condition, then there must be a continuum with no exact point at which health begins or ends. Instead of a solid and truly scientific psychiatry, we are left with a fluid system that implies that people can be half mad or half rational. According to Ey, the difference between the two worlds cannot be quantitative—a question of more or less—but is of necessity qualitative. If a person is insane, this is because an impaired organic basis prevents him from thinking or feeling like others, and prohibits interpersonal communication.

Ey does not actually deny the existence of apparently pathogenic social situations, but he does not accept the idea of 'reactive psychosis'—that is, psychosis provoked by external events. This is proven by statistics which show that psychosis does not vary according to the environment or the period: wars and revolutions do not affect its incidence. 'Everything happens exactly as though psychosis were a constant whose relation to the environment were only an incidental variable.' The real difference between the normal and the insane person is that the normal person responds to events, and is able to adjust to a change in environment, while the psychotic is not able to do so: he is never reactive. It is, of course, possible for psychosis to occur after a particular event, but this succession does not imply causality. Grief, jealousy and anxiety are everyday phenomena, and are not sufficient in themselves to explain mental illness. There is another element in the genesis of psychosis. The psychiatrist who analyses the disturbances of his patients always comes up against a 'residue' that he cannot explain, precisely because the origin of the disturbance is organic and not psychological or social. He tries to justify himself by transferring the pathological nature of the subject (the patient) on to the object (the social situation), but in vain. Faced with the same situation, the mental patient reacts differently from normal people; therefore the cause is not the situation, but the patient's organism. He reacts in a pathological way because of his particular 'heterotypy' in relation to the normal person:

> The conclusion, as we have said many a time, is that the concept of reactive psychosis is a contradiction in terms. It is true that illness always depends on life circumstances, that it is effectively inseparable from the patient's existence and particularly from the network of his relations with others; but it can never be reduced ... to the mere result of an unhappy situation. Illness depends on the threshold of response: when it occurs it is dependent on this threshold and no longer on the situation alone.

It is also true that Ey is opposed to 'organismic' interpretations. All neuroses and psychoses contain psychic elements: the patient is still related to the events in his life and his personality depends on his individual history and on the social situation in which he finds himself. However, the psychic or social elements of his personality are the part of him that remains unaffected by the illness; the fundamental source of his disturbance is elsewhere. 'If psychic causes do play a role, it remains subordinate to the role of organic disturbance.' Psychotherapy is not totally condemned, but it can only be effective to the extent that the alteration of the personality which to us may seem abnormal is not purely pathological in nature. Ey considers himself a follower of Jackson, to whom mental disorder is a phenomenon of regression and dissolution of the higher functions of the mind, due to lesions or functional disturbances of the cortical centres: illness does not create: it releases. It is the impairment of the organic infrastructure which causes a change in the mental superstructure. The error of psychoanalysis was to mistake the effect for the cause: the infantile oral, anal or narcissistic mentality which can be found in adults is not a motive force within the unconscious but the outcome of a disintegration of the adult mentality. In the same way, an emotional block can be explained by an organic injury, not by an inhibition of unconscious origin. It is impossible to imagine a more complete reversal of the sociogenetic theory. There is no need to search for such causes as social isolation, emotional deprivation, rejection, etc. These are not the real pathogenic factors; they result from or are subordinate to organic factors.

We have no reason to discuss Ey's theory in itself. I am no psychiatrist and this is not a psychiatric work. However, we must ask ourselves whether this theory, along with the genetic theory, completely bars the way to social influences or whether it allows them a place. The French sociologists Durkheim and Halbwachs were faced with a similar argument in their work on suicide, and gave the following appropriate reply:

> These are organic disorders that concern psychiatry, but at the same time all mentally-ill people are individuals who are not adjusted to their environment. Mental disorder is an element of social disequilibrium and as such concerns the science of society. . . . It is possible that among all the people with reasons for committing suicide, the ones who kill themselves are the ones who are irritable, over-sensitive and lacking in self-control. But it is no accident that they are found in greater number among professionals, industrial and business executives, and urban dwellers.

By showing variations in mental disorder according to social group, statisticians have raised a problem that cannot be solved by a theory of purely organic causation. And it will have to be solved.

This section on the place of sociogenesis in psychopathology has been in the nature of a summary of theories that either complete or contradict those presented in the first chapter. If we place these theories in confrontation, without making any choice between them, a certain number of problems emerge. We shall end this part of the chapter by listing them:

(1) It is important first of all to distinguish between neurosis and psychosis. Whereas psychosis does not vary appreciably from one period or from one society to another, neurosis is steadily increasing parallel with rapid changes in our social structure and value system. This would suggest that neurosis is more amenable than psychosis to sociological treatment. It is true that Freud's theory of the neuroses rests on a biological basis, in the sense that neurosis represents a fixation of the libido at an infantile stage of development, in particular at the Oedipal stage. But Freud demonstrates that this fixation is due to the family constellation and therefore in the final analysis to a sociological fact. Erich Fromm goes still further in the sociological line and replaces sexual rivalry in the Oedipus complex by a conflict between the child's freedom and the discipline imposed by his parents. Sullivan emphasizes interpersonal relations and Karen Horney value-conflicts. Historically speaking, sociological explanations of the origin and nature of neurosis have tended to replace biological explanations.[26] Even for psychosis, the lack of variation in the figures is not an *a priori* indication of the constitutional or organic character of the illness. Other hypotheses are possible: Goldhamer and Marshall, for example, noted that if one takes into account changes in the definition of various psychoses over time and changes in age distribution, there has been no increase in the number of psychotics in public and private hos-

pitals in Massachusetts between 1840 and 1940, although the structure of American society went through considerable upheavals between these two dates. However, they do not conclude that sociogenesis must be rejected, but they suggest that this is proof that in the causation of psychosis interpersonal relations are more important than society as a whole, these relations obviously being much more stable than the social structure.[27]

(2) A second fact emerging from this conflict of doctrines is the suggestion that the terms 'reactive neurosis' and 'reactive psychosis' have led psychiatrists on to the wrong track by placing the emphasis on situational factors. The sociologist—who is no biographer—is interested in total structures, not in events which are discrete and contingent facts—in other words, non-sociological phenomena. Here again we see the difference between the sociology of mental disorder and social psychiatry in the strictest sense. The latter discipline is primarily interested in the events that make up the history of a person, and in assessing the pathogenic quality of these events, such as an unhappy love-affair, a bereavement, a period of unemployment, etc. However, one point has been made clear: an event can only affect a person—if it does affect him at all—when it is experienced by that person. The life-history of an individual can include important collective events, such as wars and revolutions, but these collective events are only important in so far as they have a repercussion upon his consciousness, i.e. that they are 'traumas' in his life. The sociology of mental illness ignores this problem completely, since only the psychiatrist is competent to assess the importance of these traumas in the causation of psychosis and neurosis. What it is concerned with is the general 'framework' (family, institutions, etc.) within which individuals, both normal and abnormal, lead their lives. It is obvious that the effect of these general social factors (contrary to the effect of events) can only be unconscious. It is even precisely because of their unconscious nature that social causes of psychopathology have escaped the psychiatrist; the sociologist alone is capable of discovering them.

(3) We have just stated that the social framework is the same for normal and abnormal people. This introduces the problem of the relationship between the organic and the social or, alternatively, between individual disposition and environment, between psychological make-up and outside influences. The debate among psychiatrists as to whether 'events' are effective causes or merely precipitants of latent disturbances could be reopened in the sociological field. One can state simply that the sociologist does not reject hereditary factors, organic lesions and biochemical disturbances. Social factors can only operate on the individual through heredity and physiology. We do not give social factors a privileged

position and we admit that it is necessary to consider the biological side or the constitution of the individual as well as the influence of the environment. We only ask that environmental influences be recognized. This was the obvious point made by Comte: there is a correlation between phenomena of personal and social disorganization. The facts show in a striking way that mental disorder is more prevalent in areas of social disorganization than in integrated areas within a given population.[28] This cannot merely be due to chance.

(4) Up till now we have been attempting to discover whether social influences can find a place in the aetiology of mental disorder. Difficulties reappear when we try to define what we mean by 'social'. On the one hand we have the common definition applied in relation to neurosis by both traditional and modern psychoanalysts and in relation to psychosis by Goldhamer and Marshall: 'social' means anything appertaining to interpersonal relations and in particular parent-child relations in the first years of life. On the other hand, the supporters of a sociology of mental disorder define as 'social' that which relates to the whole social system. The Marxists in particular maintain that relating mental disorder to interpersonal relations is typical of 'conservatives', wrapped up in their *bourgeois* ideology, who refuse to see the class struggle as the leading factor in 'mental alienation'.[29] But here again there is a division between those who break down the social system into a series of groups and institutions (sociologists would then make a separate study of the influence of family factors, economic factors, political factors, religious factors, etc.) and those who are opposed to an analysis of particular factors and maintain that one must take an overall view of society. The first group is mainly struck by the fact that within any one society there tend to be both sick and healthy people; one should therefore begin by analysing the society to discover the pathogenic factors. The personality-environment relationship must in a sense be broken down into a series of 'variables', to be examined one by one. The second group, on the contrary, declare that the individual does not react to any one particular factor, since society is always made up of interconnected groups or institutions acting and reacting on each other to form distinctive configurations. The individual always responds to 'total situations'. The abnormal, like the normal, must be studied in its two functional dimensions, the organic and the psychological, and as part of a 'global' community and culture.[30]

We cannot at this stage reach a decision or a conclusion. Until now we have been dealing with theories only. These theories are probably based on observations and factual information, but they always comprise a set of hypotheses that go beyond the facts. We must start by giving an account of these 'facts' as they appear in the wealth of interdisciplinary empirical research which will be the subject of our next chapter. Only when we have examined the findings of this empirical research and discussed their significance will it be possible to reach a conclusion on the question of sociogenesis. But not before if we wish to avoid mingling our subjective inclinations with factual findings.

3 Can a society go mad?

Can the sociology of mental disorder be reduced to the issue of sociogenesis? Are we not running the risk of equating it with social psychiatry, which is what we wish to avoid from the very start? Is there no other possible meaning that can be given to the new science we are trying to develop in this book? If sociology is the study of collective phenomena, and if these phenomena are not equivalent to the sums of individual phenomena, would not the true sociology of mental disorder be the study of collective forms of insanity, while social psychiatry would be concerned with its individual forms? Hence the last preliminary issue remaining to be clarified: Can a society go mad? We must approach this issue step by step. First of all, we must study collective forms of mental disorder within the framework of relations between individuals, such as *folie à deux*, psychoses affecting whole households, apartment blocks, neighbourhoods and communities, on which clinical observations are available. Then we shall approach the more theoretical and hypothetical issue of deciding whether one can extend the concept of psychopathology from individuals to groups and state that societies can be neurotic, paranoid, schizophrenic, etc., as some authors maintain.

Since 1871, when Legrand du Saule introduced the concept in psychiatry of 'communicated persecution' or delusions shared by two or three people (*folie à deux* or *folie à trois*), the bibliography on the subject has become vast. It will suffice to summarize the principal stages of discovery in this field. In 1877, Lasègue and Falret discovered three conditions for the appearance of *folie à deux*. (1) Induction (contagion of insanity cannot occur unless one of the partners, the more intelligent of the two, 'induces' the psychosis). (2) Closed group (the group in which the psychosis spreads must be removed from external influences). (3) Credibility (the delusions have to retain a plausible character for others to be able to participate in them). In 1880 Régis contrasted the communication of delusions with what he called 'simultaneous insanity', which has neither active agents nor recipients: madness develops at the same time in two or more persons. This was a great step forward in that the idea of suggestibility had been dropped in favour of the recognition that the individuals involved make a personal commitment to the shared delusions, each taking an active part in their elaboration. The resulting psychosis is built up of closely interwoven personal constructions. This marks the transition from the psychology of interrelations to sociology proper. In 1900 Clérambault completed this sociology, first by recognizing that the conviction with which the recipient participates can be stronger than that of the active agent, but especially by formulating the principle of 'division of labour' in socially shared insanity: each person contributes different elements according to his constitutional make-up and personal preoccupations. Since then the original conclusions have been revised. Thus Arnaud, in contrast to Lasègue and Falret, states that in the process of induction the active partner is often less intelligent that the recipient. Delay and his collaborators found that women were more often inductive agents than men. In their article they reviewed the various contributions of their predecessors to assess whether they were validated by more recent findings. They confirmed the value of the 'closed group' principle, meaning either isolation due to a group being excluded from the rest of society (often the case with foreign families) or due to the voluntary isolation of the group following the death of the breadwinner, or financial and other difficulties. In this case the factor precipitating the psychosis is one which is crucial not to any one individual, but to the family unit as a whole. Similarly, the 'division of labour' principle seems valid: it explains why the hospitalization of one member (the one considered to be the active case) does not prevent the remaining persons from continuing in their deluded state, but on the contrary often justifies their feelings of persecution by the rest of the community (neighbours, district, etc.). On the other hand, the law of credibility is not validated, as many of the delusions found (possession by devils, for example) are clearly of a fantastic nature.[31] What we need to retain from these psychiatric studies is first of all that we are dealing with factors beyond heredity, at least in cases of transmission between husband and wife.[32] Second and more important, the division of labour has to involve, in our opinion, not only the intellectual level and the psychopathological make-up of each person concerned, but also the family structure seen in a sociological light (the nature of paternal authority, the style of parent-child relations, and the models of behaviour prescribed by society). The psychosis follows the patterns of interpersonal relations in a closed setting, exhibiting the particular conflicts and tensions created by these patterns.

However, psychosis can also spread to a wider group, or at least to a wider circle than the family. Heuyer studied a case of delusions involving five people: the instigators were a fourteen-year-old boy who built up a whole world of imaginary noises and his mother; they were joined first by the rest of their household and then by the whole neighbourhood. Heuyer was able to classify socially-shared psychosis into cases involving next-door neighbours, apartment blocks and neighbourhoods.[33] This brings us to 'mass insanity', involving even larger groups: we shall return to this question later. Note, however, that in this instance also the delusion spreads along particular lines according to the structure of the community; in other words, it happens within a certain social framework which predetermines its course and its limits.

Nevertheless we are still dealing with cases of simultaneous disturbance. In connection with the pathology of the family, psychoanalysis has brought to light another form of socially transmitted disorder: contagion from one generation to another. As Margaret Mead says, anxious parents create anxious children, who grow up to produce an anxious society, which in turn creates even more anxious parents. We return by a different route to socially shared insanity. But we must be careful: the agency here is not heredity, but the learning process. Neurotic conflicts are taught by the parents and learned by the children.[34] We have sufficiently emphasized in another book the learning of morbid patterns through the family and socialization[35] for it to be unnecessary to return to this topic. There is a case, in fact, for looking at trans-mission through learning according to whether the kinship system is patrilineal or matrilineal, to bring out its characteristics more clearly. Let us conclude that the process of contagion from the individual to the group can take two forms: simultaneous psychosis and propagation over time (from one generation to another) of fundamental emotional disturbance, which we could call by analogy with the first term 'consecutive psychosis'.

Beside these shared psychoses that still only affect small groups of people there are mass psychoses that spread by contagion in convents, through the countryside, from village to village, reaching in some cases considerable numbers of people.[36] With mass in-sanity we are still within the same sociological field on which the studies of simultaneous insanity are based: the sociology of inter-action (and not of the collective mind):

The cumulative intensity of irrational communications can be observed throughout the ages: it reaches its peak in the phenomena known as mass psychoses. The impetus comes from one individual whose behaviour was previously irregular or is only suddenly recognized as such, due to a particular configuration of social events or conflicts. This impetus can be considerably strengthened by the association of the first agent

with a second agent electively receptive to the first. Because
of this reciprocal process, they constitute a pathogenic couple:
witch and inquisitor, possessed and exorcisor, epileptic and
nurse, unstable person and mental defective. Contagion spreads
from person to person, relayed by similar relationships which are
always present in any community. In every case the drama is
played out on the level of these relationships.[37]

The same principles apply as in *folie à deux*, which is in fact a
stage in the creation of mass psychosis; induction, division of
labour, even closed *milieu* (though the epidemic spreads to a
larger number of people). The birth of communication media, such
as radio, television, or even newspapers, complicates the phenomenon by enlarging it still further, but it does not essentially alter
the process. A good example of this is Orson Welles's programme
on the Martian invasion.[38] There has been a great deal of interest in
mass psychosis especially when it is of a mystical nature, such as
the epidemics of demonic possession from the Middle Ages to the
seventeenth century, the mass terrors of the year 1000 or of the
French Revolution, bizarre religious sects, Messianic movements,
or 'liberation cults', as Lanternari calls them, etc. There are
valuable monographs available on all these phenomena, written
by historians, anthropologists, or psychiatrists, but, with the exception of Messianism, there are very few truly sociological studies.
Now, these phenomena cannot be explained simply by mental
contagion; to understand them one must draw on political,
economic and even linguistic sources. We call attention in this context to Certeau's work on the possessed people of Loudun.[39] He
shows that this phenomenon of demonic possession must be seen in
the context of the whole of French society; it is necessary to go
beyond a merely psychopathological determinism which can only
provide a superficial and fragmentary picture. Some contemporary
psychiatrists are very much aware of this necessity. For example,
Deshaies writes:

> Phenomena known as mass psychosis and neurosis certainly
> do not represent autonomous and specific forms of illness. . . .
> Rumours, panic, destructive rage and fanatical states manifested
> by crowds are collective movements in which the individual
> is carried away and submerged. . . . The word 'pathology' in this
> context is not justified, nor the word 'social', unless it be by
> an unfortunate metaphor.[40]

It could not be better put.
In fact, the same deceptive term has been applied to widely
different and often diametrically opposite manifestations. Let us

list a few. First of all there are those movements which may of course attract psychotics, but which are not inherently morbid; on the contrary, they are normal responses to frustrating social situations, and they also have useful functions. These are the Messianic movements. They sometimes involve, as in the case of the Cargo cult, a distortion of reality, but it is not a noticeably different distortion from that of myths and folk-beliefs; in fact, its roots are to be found there. A second set of phenomena, such as the *tarantella* in Italy,[41] are more markedly psychopathological in character. But it is not possible to use the term 'mass insanity' here either, since we are dealing with a traditional model dictated by a particular cultural *milieu*, the accepted group model of the 'proper way to go mad', which is imposed on anyone in a state of crisis. The third set of phenomena are those described by Deshaies, whom we quoted above: general panic, bouts of mass aggression, etc., what used to be known as the *folie des foules*, or crowd-madness, a fashionable notion at the time of Sighèle or Le Bon. The use of the term *folie* implies a belief in a collective mind over and above the individual. If the individual mind can be impaired by mental illness, why not then, by analogy, the collective mind? The irrational movements of crowds are indeed provoked by a loss of social control and the eruption of instinctual impulses. This can be compared to the resurgence of lower forms of mental activity when higher cerebral activities are inhibited or eliminated; but here again we are dealing with an analogy rather than a homology. It may be possible here to speak of 'social pathology', but certainly not of pathology in the psychiatric sense and social in the sociological sense, since in effect the social framework is disrupted and social controls removed: it is the antithesis of the Durkheimian definition of collective conscience.

Now that we have cleared the ground, what remains? First of all, we have the occurrence of collective neurosis induced by a violent trauma experienced by several persons at once, but without any definite evidence of communication or contagion. The best-known case is that of the handful of American sailors at Guadalcanal in August 1942 who were subjected to such a degree of mental and physical stress that the whole group suffered a neurotic break-down. Once the stress was removed the majority recovered without treatment. Secondly, we have collective neurosis or psychosis brought about through transmission of delusions in couples or through networks of persons acting as relay-points, e.g. mystical and demonic epidemics. In our opinion, only a sociological approach can explain the formation of these couples, indicate the patterns of interconnection and show how the relay-points emerge. We are left with the final question whether society itself can become insane. This question never occurred to the early psychiatrists, but since the appearance of Fascism and Nazism the issue has become a crucial one.

The idea that a society can be 'sane' or 'sick' clashes with our definition of normal as adjusted: if people are adjusted to a sick society, then they will all be neurotics. According to Erich Fromm, just as mental disorder can involve two people, so it can involve millions. This makes the diagnosis of collective insanity difficult, since it affects the whole of society, including the psychiatrist. However it is undeniable that our present society is pathological from a psychiatric point of view.[42] Devereux, inspired by the work of Bain and Burrow, also formulated the idea of social neurosis. This idea obviously implies that the person who introjects the norms and values of society will be neurotic, and that it is not the individual who must be treated, but the society. The rebel in this case, the non-adjusted person, is the sane one.[43] As was the case in Nazi Germany, all oppressive minorities on taking power demand that the oppressed should not only adjust to their frustrating situation, but also manifest a distinctive form of neurosis. At the same time the majority develops a symmetrical neurosis: 'The alloplastic efforts of the oppressors produce autoplastic manifestations of equal or greater intensity than the manifestations imposed on the oppressed', with the final result that the whole society becomes neurotic.

Obviously the statement that society is mad rather than the individual does not mean that the collective mind is affected by psychiatric disorder: neurosis and psychosis are always individual phenomena. What it does mean is that society magnifies the morbid tendencies of its members: it creates situations that have the effect of increasing the numbers of mentally-ill people. In fact, we are merely dealing with a particular case of sociogenesis as described above. It is important not to confuse the sociological with the psychiatric meaning of the word 'pathology'; what happens is that phenomena of social pathology bring about a growth of psychopathological phenomena. This takes us back to Comte's original idea, which we shall deal with later in our discussion of empirical research. Other ideas can also be connected with the concept of social pathology. Thomas M. Feuch, for example (*Social Conflict and Psychic Conflict*), while keeping the two phenomena separate, shows how social conflicts can involve great numbers of people with psychic conflicts that are either latent or overt. These psychic conflicts add up to produce mass delusions and mass phobias (such as the fear of Communism in the U.S.A.) similar to those encountered by the psychiatrist.

This seems a valid point of view. Some authors have gone further still. Trigant Burrow (*The Social Neurosis*) mentions hysterical societies with organized defence mechanisms, disturbances of language (metonymy), reversion to childhood fantasies, etc. Ruth Benedict (*Patterns of Culture*) speaks of paranoid societies. This is a step beyond the sociogenetic approach; it is a full acceptance of the idea that our societies can become 'insane' in the same way as individuals, and that these collective insanities can be fitted into the categories of clinical psychopathology (hysteria, paranoia, etc.). This idea can take several forms. It can be a simple extension to society as a whole of the concept of interpersonal relations: when a head of state or a particularly powerful leader is mentally ill, he can—by contagion or interpsychic communication—transmit his disturbance to his whole people. This is the way Hitler was frequently viewed in the U.S.A.[44] The other form this idea can take—as typified by René Laforgue's book *Talleyrand* (a psychoanalysis of the French mind)—is the assumption that the collective mind obeys exactly the same laws as the individual psyche.[45] Personally, we do not agree that it is possible to equate collective phenomena with individual processes, and we would tend to agree with authors like Alexander, who do not believe that one can 'psychoanalyse' societies.[46] We have explained why elsewhere.[47] The disorders of society can bear some resemblance to individual disorders, but to go any further and to speak in terms of hysterical societies or paranoid cultures is sheer word-play. We will conclude this chapter with the remark that there is such a thing as a sociology of mental disorder, but there is no such thing as 'psychiatric sociology', a point which had to be made in order to clear up any confusion before we proceed further.

IV From ecology to the study of communities

1 Town and country

It has been noted for a long time that there is more mental disorder in towns than in the country.[1] For example, the 1940 figures for the U.S.A. give the following rates:

Table 3 Diagnostic category and ratio of town- to country-dwellers in the U.S.A.

Diagnostic category	Ratio of town- to country-dwellers
Senile psychosis	2 to 1
Arteriosclerotic psychosis	2·5 to 1
General paresis	2·6 to 1
Alcoholic psychosis	2·6 to 1
Manic-depressive psychosis	1·3 to 1
Dementia praecox	1·8 to 1

It was, of course, easy to explain this difference in terms of the contrast between the affective, personal and intimate relationships of country life and the impersonal almost purely contractual ones of large cities, between traditional organic communities and the mechanical nature of contacts between people, or anomie. One

78

could blame the disappearance in the city of the extended family and the controlling influence of the village, the increasingly stressful and competitive nature of urban life, the isolation of the individual, etc. It is a well-known picture and it is unnecessary for us to describe it at length.

But first we must point out that from the sociological point of view the city is not a homogeneous entity. Clearly, country people moving to the town tend to experience difficulties in adjusting to a new environment, and these difficulties can have pathological results. However, there are also great numbers of people born in the city of city-dwelling parents, and who therefore do not have any adjustment problems. Similarly, rural areas do not all present the same picture. For example, in the Côte d'Or Département, melancholia is more frequent in the richer plains than in the poorer mountainous regions, which require a more stubborn and painstaking effort from the peasant.[2] We must replace these generalities about town and country by more specific and precise statements that take into account the diversity of geographical settings and of social structure. The most important point is that all the early studies maintaining that the country is more favourable to mental health than the metropolis are based on first admissions to mental hospitals. This leads us to wonder whether the high urban rate of mental disorder is not due to the fact that, first, towns offer better hospital facilities, and, second, that cramped urban living conditions do not allow for the home care of disturbed persons: it is much easier to look after a mental defective, a neurotic or even some types of psychotic in an isolated farmhouse.[3] Moreover, popular conceptions are very different in the two settings: insanity is not regarded as a stigma in the city, and with the progress of medicine there is a growing belief in the possibility of cure if the sick person is treated as soon as he shows signs of disturbance. This means in fact that statistics based on first admissions give the 'degree of tolerance' shown by urban and rural populations towards the mentally ill rather than the actual frequency of psychosis or psychoneurosis among town- or country-dwellers. However, we cannot, on the basis of this hypothesis, reject *a priori* the idea that the city does not constitute a more highly pathogenic environment than the country. Among Army conscripts rejected each year on psychiatric grounds there are always more town- than country-dwellers. So we still have not solved the problem.

To obtain the true picture, psychiatrists and sociologists must either, if the population is small enough, interview everyone in a particular community (as Lin did in Formosa, where he tested and interviewed 19,913 people), or, if the population is too large, use sampling methods and generalize from the data gathered for the rest of the area. A third approach is to make a comparative study of first admissions to hospitals in towns and of all the individuals, farm by farm, in a rural area. Thus Lin compared a country area of Formosa, a small village and a district of a large town; he found no significant differences except for a slightly higher rate of schizophrenia in the urban area and of mental deficiency and senile psychosis in the rural areas.[4] Alexander Leighton, as mentioned above, has recently been engaged with others on a vast survey, the Stirling County Study of Psychiatric Disorder and Sociocultural Environment, in Bristol, an American town of 3,000 inhabitants, and in the neighbouring countryside. He used a special questionnaire designed to detect personality disorders that had escaped the attention of doctors and mental hospitals. So far it appears that the most important factor is not demographic concentration, but the degree of organization or disorganization of social life, the latter being found in both rural and urban areas.

This is the crucial point. We have inherited from Rousseau an idyllic conception of country life; however, there are rural problem areas as well as urban ones. Certain features of city life have been exaggerated, such as mobility and the impersonality of social relations, while these same features have been overlooked in the country. Large American cities harbour religious or ethnic communities that are stable and harmonious, while cases of rural anomie exist among mobile agricultural workers, as in the California so well depicted by American novelists.[5] This is equally true for Europe, with its isolated regions, areas of agricultural underdevelopment and declining villages where only a few hardened and frustrated families remain. Let us give a few examples.

Table 4 Morbidity rate by diagnostic category in a Norwegian fishing village

	Number	Rate per 1,000
Schizophrenia	6	4·5
Manic-depressive psychosis	2	1·5
Total number of psychotics	38	28·7
Number of people showing disturbance (psychotic or non-psychotic)	212	160·0

Bremer made a study of a small fishing village in the Arctic region of Norway from 1939 to 1944. He found that in a population of 1,325 one person out of every five showed signs of maladjustment, which in half the cases amounted to mental disorder. Table 4 summarizes his findings.

Böök studied a rural area of northern Sweden with a population of 8,931. He found 364 cases of mental disorder from 1902 to 1949, of whom 85 were schizophrenic (9·6 per 1,000 population) and only two manic depressives (0·2 per 1,000 population). All the schizophrenics were catatonic.[6] We will not attempt to discover at present whether these high rates are due, as Böök maintains, to genetic factors, with isolation forcing people to intermarry and thus to transmit 'pathological genes', or whether, as Bremer thinks, social factors need to be considered, such as the lack of contact with the outside world, the low economic status of the inhabitants, and the disruption of families following the German occupation of the area. The relevant point is this: when, instead of looking at hospitalization figures, an intensive study is made of a small, isolated agricultural or fishing community, the idyllic picture according to which country people are better preserved from mental disorder than city-dwellers is shown to be entirely false. The rate of schizophrenia that Böök found is one of the highest ever recorded. Although Mayer-Gross used a different technique (the British do not readily submit to psychiatric examination), that of questioning the leaders of the community, he obtained an equally significant picture for a rural area of Scotland.[7]

Table 5 Morbidity rate by diagnostic category in a rural area of Scotland (1948)

	Number	Rate per 1,000
Schizophrenia	230	4·2
Manic-depressive psychosis	199	3·5
Psychosis	1,225	21·8
Total cases of abnormality	5,105	90·0
Total population	56,000	—

French psychiatrists, who are fairly hostile to statistics, but keen to understand the phenomena in depth with the aid of case studies, have given the best analyses we know of psychosis in rural settings. It is true that at first they tended mainly to blame alcoholism. In wine-producing regions, such as Chablis, or cider regions, such as Le Puisay, Scherer discovered a high frequency of alcoholic psychosis. However, the use of alcohol in itself is only the effect of more fundamental causes of a sociological order. At the 1950 International Congress of Criminology in Paris, Tosquellier drew attention to the chain reaction operating in certain villages of the Lozère region that are in rapid decline. The head of the family reacts against social disorganization either by becoming withdrawn or by becoming involved in politics; he tends to be paranoid and his wife is generally anxious. The second son of such a couple remains emotionally immature and dependent on his mother. He is often a sexual offender and shows an embryonic form of schizophrenia. Full-blown schizophrenia develops in the next generation in the eldest son, who often escapes from an intolerable situation to work in the town. Scherer, on the other hand, attributes rural psychosis to isolation. He gives many typical examples of this. We find the elderly couple, two bachelors or a brother and sister, living on a desolate farm, trying to drown their emotional frustration in mechanical and aimless work, and weaving delusions on incestuous themes or based on guilt. Then there are the children suddenly loaded with too much responsibility on the death of the father. Or the situation where several families live under one roof to avoid dividing the property, with all the possibilities of conflict this entails; the patriarch stifles the young people's ambitions and creates brooding resentment often conducive to neurosis. Meanwhile, as he grows old, he tends to develop delusions of persecution arising from a fear of being deprived of his authority. In the final analysis it is the present structure of agricultural society in France, especially in isolated regions, which explains the psychoses typical of rural life. Scherer concludes with a quotation from Hesnard: 'Psychosis often appears not when there is a severing of internal family or tribal links, but, on the contrary, where the abnormal rigidity of these presocial links prevents the individual from becoming free from the authority of his family or of his restricted group which has remained cut off from the rest of society.'[8]

Obviously the issue becomes clearer and the contradictions disappear when, instead of drawing an ecological comparison between town and country, we study rural or urban communities with reference to their degree of social organization or disorganization. The disorganized village can be just as responsible for neurosis and psychosis as certain neighbourhoods of our large cities.

One should not conclude, however, that rural areas are less conducive to mental health, for so long as the village remains a living organism rather than an ossified and archaic structure, so long as it does not lose its soul, it can remain impermeable to mental disorder. Scherer gives the example of certain Dutch settlements in France that have kept a strong and harmonious community life: they are apparently quite immune to psychiatric disorder.

What is the secret of these self-sufficient and immune rural communities, like oases of mental health in the midst of the countryside? Scherer confines himself to a statement of fact without taking his research any further. But in the U.S.A. we find similar 'oases' which have been the object of psychiatric studies: the Hutterite communities.[9]

The Hutterites are an Anabaptist sect who emigrated from Russia to Canada and the U.S.A. between 1874 and 1877. They live cut off from the 'world', which they regard as sinful, on collective farms or colonies, of which there are over ninety. Each colony is composed of about sixteen family units, with a leader and a minister appointed by the community. For a long time they were considered to be completely immune to mental illness. The reasons given were that the social cohesiveness of the colonies protected the individual against insecurity, poverty, illness and other stresses and strains of living, and that religious values fostered this social cohesiveness. However, Eaton and Weil, who studied nineteen of these colonies in depth and visited the others several times, did in fact find mental disorders, namely:

Table 6 Morbidity rate by diagnostic category in the Hutterite communities

	Number	Rate per 1,000
Schizophrenia	9	1
Manic-depressive psychosis	39	4·6
Total psychotics	53	6·2
Total mentally ill	199	23·2
Total population	8,542	—

The most striking fact is the small number of schizophrenics—one of the lowest rates known—whose symptoms are in fact relatively mild. This explains why the Hutterites were thought to be free from mental illness owing to their social and cultural cohesiveness. On the other hand, we find a very high rate of manic-depressive reactions; for the Hutterites depression is not in fact an illness, but a normal phenomenon, a 'temptation by the devil', like the trials God sent to Job. This means that psychotics remain integrated into the group (while being relieved of their responsibilities during their breakdown). Thus their existence escaped the attention of the first psychiatrists who took an interest in the Hutterites. Later on we shall see how this phenomenon can be explained when we study the influence of religion in mental illness; it is enough to emphasize here that Hutterite culture does not give more protection against personality disorders than any other culture.

The concept of neurosis is also foreign to the Hutterite mind, but this does not mean that their people are free from it. Eaton and Weil diagnosed 33 cases per 1,000, mainly women; the Hutterites classified them as organically ill. Kaplan and Plaut, who administered the T.A.T. to Hutterites, also found, beneath the apparent harmony and stability of the group, many unresolved problems, hidden pockets of repressed aggression and deep-seated anxiety connected with the aggressive tendencies condemned by Hutterite culture. The authors acknowledge the fact that these problems do not usually produce severe symptoms. Hutterite culture accepts the individual in a state of crisis, tries to reduce his practical, economic and psychological difficulties as much as possible, encourages him to play a responsible part in the community and surrounds him with active sympathy (mainly in the form of prayer, attentiveness and nurture), thus forming a sort of therapeutic group that reduces manifestations of mental disorder to a minimum. The general conclusion emerging from the study of these settlements that have shut themselves away from 'worldly' temptations is that social cohesion does not rule out psychiatric disorder, but does play an effective role, either therapeutically or preventively, in reducing tension and avoiding social alienation.

Rural psychiatry is one of the most rewarding fields of research in the sociology of mental disorder. We have seen that by progressing from purely demographic or ecological factors (concentration or dispersal of the population) to the sociological study of rural communities, taking into account their structure and their values, things become more complicated, and the early conclusions of the ecologists have to be revised or at least qualified. Problems and stress creating neurosis can be found everywhere, and no society is immune from psychosis. But some environmental settings, such as regions with rural problems, are more conducive to the development of mental disorder, while others, such as harmonious and thriving villages, tend to limit its severity. So there is no point in talking about the country in general, nor in assuming on the basis of the origin of hospitalized patients that there is a universally valid relationship between mental disorder and urban or rural habitat. The social structures of isolated, dying villages in the mountains is different from that of prosperous villages in the plains; wine-producing regions that remain individualistic in spite of the co-operative system are different from the Norman *bocage* and the moors of Brittany, to mention only France. What is more, these structures change over time; there are underdeveloped areas and areas of progressive agriculture. We must distinguish between regions with large estates often employing foreign farm labourers (Poles, Spaniards, etc.) who are more or less relegated to the margins of French society, and whose work is alienated and alienating, and regions of small holdings where the farms are either scattered or grouped in villages. Each region has its particular features, a fact which was first brought to light by Vidal de la Blanche's 'human geography', and which could provide a framework for intensive studies by psychiatrists in collaboration with psychologists and sociologists or rural anthropologists. Mental-health maps of the French départements have been drawn up in the past, but they are based on hospitalization figures that are inevitably unrepresentative. They ought to be constructed in the same way as Boulard and Le Bras's maps of religious practices, from painstaking studies parish by parish. Comprehensive surveys or at least studies using sampling techniques are needed to clarify the many apparently ambiguous links between different rural social structures and personality disorders. In this way regions would emerge, each with its particular psychiatric characteristics, obviously related to geographical, economic, political and social factors. It would admittedly be a long and exacting task, which is probably why we know much more at present about urban than rural psychiatry.

2 Urban ecological areas and the distribution of mental disorder in the towns

Ecology is the study of human relations as influenced by the physical environment—which means that it does not study social relations as such, but symbiotic relations. One of the most important concepts this discipline has produced is the idea of segregation or localization of urban populations in separate areas as a result of competition: wealthy areas, working-class areas, immigrant areas, suburbs, etc.

But these areas are not permanent: invasions or penetrations by populations originally from another area can occur—for example, a white area can be penetrated by Negroes. But the invasion that interests us here is the one brought about by the encroachment of the centre of the city, the business and entertainment district, upon the residential areas. The result of this is that people leave their home, rents fall, a transient zone of hotels and rooming-houses grows up, slums develop, the area becomes a meeting-ground for prostitutes, riff-raff, recent immigrants, etc.; in fact, a whole area of social and family disorganization is created. If the sociological argument can be applied to psychiatric phenomena, this is the very place one would expect to find the greatest number of mentally-ill people. Do the facts confirm this prediction?

From his observations in Chicago, Burgess found he could divide the city into five concentric zones: (1) the central or business district; (2) the zone in transition, gradually encroached upon by the first, which we have called the zone of disorganization; (3) the zone of working-men's homes; (4) the wealthy residential zone; and (5) the suburbs, with their population of commuters who work in town and only return home at night. Burgess's followers, often known as the 'Chicago School', discovered a law governing the relationship between social problems and the concentric zones of the city: the greatest concentration of social problems is found in the second zone and there is a gradual decline towards the periphery. Shaw gives the following figures for juvenile delinquency (this phenomenon follows the same curve as the number of families on relief and the number of immigrants, and is inversely related to the number of owner-occupiers).

Table 7 Juvenile delinquency and ecological areas in Chicago

	Zone in transition	2-mile radius	3-mile radius	4-mile radius	5-mile radius
Delinquency rate	37·0	15·6	7·2	2·6	1·6
Families on relief	4·7	2·4	1·5	0·25	0·3
Foreign-born heads of families	51·5	40·3	38·3	27·5	25·5
Families owning homes	4·5	11·3	25·5	33·0	41·0

Diagram 2 Rate of mental disorders in Chicago (1930–1) per 100,000 adults (1930 population) (from Faris and Dunham)

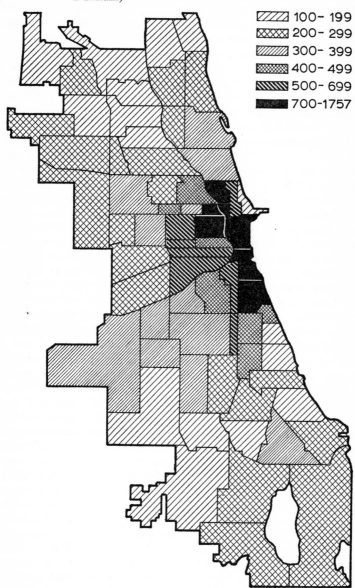

Mowrer drew attention to the variation in family type from one area to another: emancipated families that are isolated and removed from social control in the zone in transition, father-dominated and even patriarchal families in the working-class areas and particularly in immigrant communities, such as the Jewish ghetto or Little Sicily, egalitarian families in the middle-class areas and, finally, mother-dominated families in the suburbs, where the wife reigns in the absence of the husband, who is there only at night. Here also family disorganization, characterized by desertion and divorce, follows the same law of progressive decrease from the centre to the periphery. Walter Reckless found the following pattern for prostitution: a brothel area corresponding to the zone in transition, an area of undercover prostitution in the adjacent rooming-house area, the disappearance of prostitution in the low- and high-income residential areas, and its reappearance, but only after the automobile had become fashionable, in the suburbs: the prostitution of the well-to-do.[10] We could give unlimited examples of this regularity. The present few suffice to show, at least for Chicago, the rule of progressive decrease in social problems from the centre of the town to the periphery. We now need to see whether mental disorder shows the same regularity. Faris and Dunham found the following pattern for first admissions to public and private mental hospitals in Chicago: from the centre extending towards the south, the zone rates (per 100,000 population) were 362, 337, 175, 115, 88, 74, 71, and from the centre to the north-west, 362, 177, 95, 71, 66, 55. This appears to confirm the rule of progressive decrease. But further analysis shows that this is mainly valid for schizophrenia; manic-depressive psychosis does not show this regularity, but is distributed randomly throughout the city. As for schizophrenia, it reaches its highest peak in the area of social disorganization (centre and hobo area, 1,195; Negro area, 514; wealthy areas, 111). But it takes on different forms in different areas: the paranoid and hebephrenic types predominate in the areas of greatest mobility where there are many hotels and rooming-houses, while the catatonic type is found in the immigrant and Negro areas. Organic psychoses follow the same regular pattern as functional psychoses: the rate of psychosis caused by alcohol and narcotic drugs drops from 554 to 10 from the centre to the periphery; general paralysis also shows the highest rate in the area of social disorganization; the senile psychosis rate decreases from 35 in the apartment-house district to 0·8 in the area of small individual suburban houses, and psychosis due to arteriosclerosis also drops, from 134·4 to 2·9. The pattern is too pronounced and too regular to be due to chance. However, as a control, Faris and Dunham chose a small town on Rhode Island, Providence. There are no real slums to be found

Diagram 3   Sub-communities based on census tracts of Chicago. Rate of mental disorders (1922–34) according to the zones and divisions of the city (per 100,000 population aged fifteen and over)

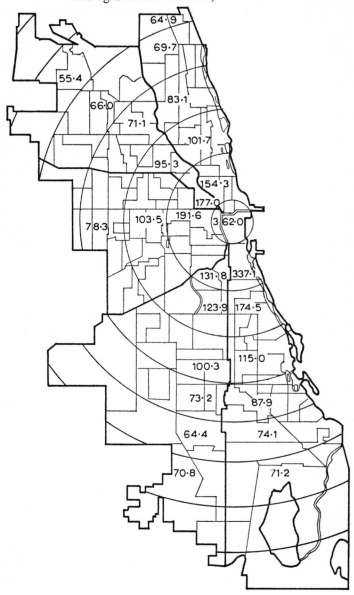

there, but the town can be divided into two parts, the old and the newly built areas. It is in the area of decaying apartment-houses that they found the highest rate of mental disorder, particularly of schizophrenia. From the old part to the modern area the same decreasing trend is present; starting with a rate of 105 or more, we find progressively: 70–104·99, 35–69·99; finally, 34·99 and under (per 100,000 population).[11]

Thus Faris and Dunham were confident that they had discovered a universal rule. The regularities cannot be attributed to poverty, since first admissions to the wealthier nursing-homes have been included. What is more, if poverty were responsible, we should find a similar distribution for all disorders, whereas we have seen that different types of illness predominate in different areas. We must also rule out the possibility of statistical error due to the very great mobility of the population in the areas of disorganization (Ross noted in 1933 a complete population turnover every three or four months),[12] because even after corrections have been made to eliminate the transient population, the mental illness rate in the hobo area is still higher than in the rest of the town. On the other hand, we may well wonder, as Burgess did in his Preface to Faris and Dunham's book, whether the high rate of mental disorder in the area of disorganization is not due to people who are already disturbed moving there to escape into anonymity and isolation. The authors did not think so, first because manic-depressive psychotics are not found in this zone, and next because the age distribution in the zone shows a greater concentration of young than old patients. Personality disorders would thus be caused by the living conditions of certain areas, the breaking up of family ties, loneliness, the disappearance of all social control and all opportunities for social interaction. In fact, there are certain urban areas that destroy mental health.

Faris and Dunham's pioneer study—which quickly became a classic—was the point of departure for a whole series of investigations in the U.S.A. (we shall come to the French studies later), some confirming their findings and others contradicting them. About ten years later Mowrer took up the study of the distribution of mental disorder in Chicago, and found that the same regularities applied to toxic psychosis and general paresis.[13] Queen compared the results of research done between the first Chicago study and the Second World War in six large American cities. He reached the conclusion that even if the results do not always agree, at least in two of the towns—Columbus, studied by McKenzie, and Seattle, studied by Lind and Schmidt—there is a similar distribution to that found in Chicago.[14] Dunham himself came back to the problem in 1955, prompted by Schröder's work.[15] He concluded that his hypothesis of the concentration of mental disorder in the centre of the town and the decline towards the periphery remained valid.[16] But there have also been investigations reaching opposite conclusions. For example, in St Louis no pattern was found at all either for manic-depressive psychosis or for schizophrenia.[17] In Milwaukee, as opposed to Chicago, manic-depressive psychosis was not distributed at random, but was concentrated in the downtown area.[18] But these different results are only apparently chaotic; a contradiction exists only if the model of concentric zones is a universal model, yet we know that there are many different types of city and that ecological patterns can vary. The issue is not so much to prove the existence of a rule as to see whether or not particular disorders are concentrated in particular zones. If there are in fact variations in ecological pattern from one town to another, and if there is a correlation between psychiatric and ecological factors, then we shall naturally have different patterns from town to town, without the ecological theory being in any way invalidated.

This is why we agree with Belknap and Jaco when they chose to study, in contrast to Chicago, a commercial-industrial city, Austin, Texas, a political and administrative capital.[19] The pattern of the incidence of psychosis is very different from the one found by Faris and Dunham: there is a high rate of disturbance in the centre, but the rate is also high in the satellite communities around the capital. However, if we exclude manic-depressive cases, senile psychosis, general paresis and cerebral arteriosclerosis, the rates are lower than in the rest of the U.S.A.:

Table 8 Comparison of mental disorder rates in Austin, Chicago and the U.S.A.

	(1946–52, rate per 100,000 population)		
	Austin	*Chicago*	*U.S.A.*
Total rate of disorders	44·7	—	70·8
Schizophrenia	16·1	36·8	22·7
Manic-depressive psychosis	11·4	8·0	5·8

European research has been more interested in the study of communities than in specifically ecological studies. Chombart de Lauwe showed that in such a city as Paris it is possible to distinguish concentric zones (the heart of Paris, the acculturation or melting-pot zone with its various nationalities or classes, which corresponds to the American zone in transition, the zone of peripheral *arrondissements*, the industrial zone, the inner suburbs, the outer suburbs, and the outskirts which are still semi-rural). But these zones are less meaningful than other types of division: the *bourgeois* west, the proletarian east, and between the two, on the right bank, the centre.[20] Unfortunately, it is difficult to base an ecological analysis of mental disorder in Paris on this particular pattern, since we do not have any data on private nursing-homes, but only on State mental hospitals; only part of the population would be represented—namely, the poorer classes. However, we do have an excellent study by Mme Chombart de Lauwe (*Psychopathologie de l'Enfant Inadapté*, published by the C.N.R.S.) giving data for children under fourteen, excluding mental defectives and children with organic disturbances. Psychological disorders are concentrated in certain areas of Paris, either in the melting-pot areas (which are also the acculturation and rooming-house areas) or in the socio-economically deprived areas. In Bordeaux, which was used for purposes of comparison, the greatest concentration of maladjusted children was also found in the under-privileged areas (the map of broken homes and the map of psychological disturbance coincide perfectly), while delinquent children are concentrated in the areas of old and overcrowded dwellings, low economic status and high rate of unemployment. Thus both in France and the U.S.A. we find urban areas that are pathological and equally regular distributions of mental disorder.

The ecological factor that appears to be the most important according to recent studies is population density—probably more so than the segregation of the population according to economic status. Gruenberg found that rates of senile dementia were highest in areas of overcrowding (Onondaga region, Syracuse, U.S.A.):

More than 2·25 persons per room: 395·3 per 100,000 population
Less than 1·25 persons per room: 213·2 per 100,000 population[21]

We do not deny that ecological factors can operate to produce a higher rate of senile psychosis or psychosis due to arteriosclerosis, but the difference in rates found by Gruenberg could well be due to the fact that it is difficult to keep disturbed old people in small flats. However, Mme Chombart de Lauwe found at the other extreme of the age-scale, among children living in low-rent municipal housing, a 'danger threshold' for overcrowding of between 2 and 2·5 people per room (between 8 and 10 sq. m. of floorspace per person):

Table 9 Psychic disturbance in children and number of persons per room

	Less than two persons per room, %	Two or more persons per room, %
Aggressive behaviour	35·2	64·8
Stealing, truancy	33·3	66·7
Nervous symptoms	43	57
Psychomotor disturbances	49	51

Diagram 4 Distribution of three groups of mental disorder in some areas of Paris. Chronic disorders 1948 and 1950 (men and women)

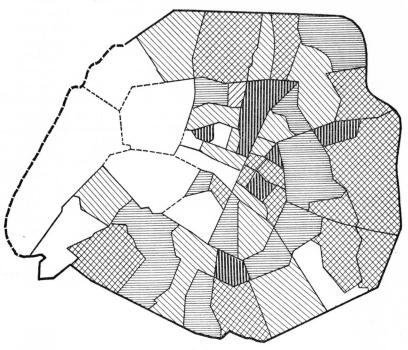

	3 and over per 10,000 population
	2–2·99 „ „ „
	1·25–1·99 „ „ „
	0·01–1·24 „ „ „
	0 „ „ „
----	Boundary of *arrondissement* not included in study.

G. Mayer-Massé, *Monographie de l'Institut National d'Hygiène, Études de Socio-psychiatrie*, No. 7, Paris, 1955, p. 38.

Diagram 5 Distribution of three groups of mental disorder in some areas of Paris and some communes of the Seine Département. Chronic Disorders 1948 and 1950 (Men and Women)

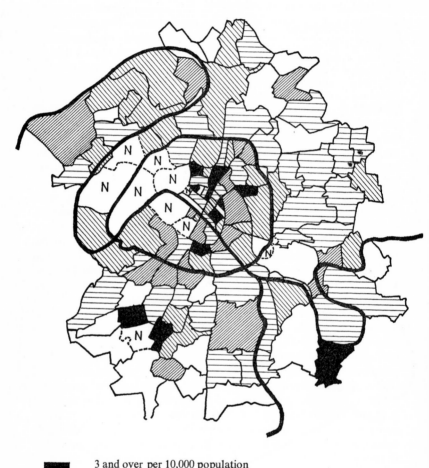

	3 and over per 10,000 population
	2–2·99 ,, ,, ,,
	1·25–1·99 ,, ,, ,,
	0·01–1·24 ,, ,, ,,
	0 ,, ,, ,,
- - - - -	Boundary of area not included in study.

G. Mayer-Massé, *Monographie de l'Institut National d'Hygiène, Études de Socio-psychiatrie*, No. 7, Paris, 1955.

Obviously the child living in a flat where his exploratory activities are limited, where he is frequently restricted and physically punished because he tires or irritates his parents, will be more prone to emotional disturbance. On the other hand there appears to be a 'threshold of equilibrium' (between 14 and 16 sq. m. per person), and between the two thresholds an intermediary zone where the distribution of disorders is more or less random. The principle of a 'danger threshold' can equally apply to the study of disorders in adults; the building of high-density housing estates makes this an urgent problem. Several studies are being made in France at present; the results appear to contradict each other so far, because the variables have not all been controlled. Some investigators, such as Le Guillant, have been struck by an increase in problems, the least severe of these being incipient neurosis in certain suburbs of Paris. Others have found the opposite to be true in the large estates of the suburbs of Toulouse. However, these investigators have usually been sociologists working alone and not as part of a team including psychiatrists or psychologists, and they therefore base their conclusions on the overt content of oral responses. It will be some time yet before we can hope for precise and clear-cut findings to emerge.

Ecological methods. The application of ecological methods to the study of mental disorder has been criticized. Criticisms from the statistical angle, such as those of Ross,[22] need not detain us here. It may be true that there are no significant differences between the rates of mental illness in different communities, nor indices refined enough to measure the specific conditions of each area. Nevertheless, the majority of the rates are significantly different from area to area within any one city, and this remains valid even though cities may present different patterns. This is not the most important problem. Ecological studies show clearly that particular types of illness are concentrated in particular areas. But does the area have a pathogenic effect *per se*? Or should one look for other factors? It is understandable that bad housing conditions can contribute to neurosis, but can they also explain psychosis and in particular schizophrenia? According to Faris and Dunham, the ecological area is important in itself. They saw, for example, in the isolation of white people in Negro communities and in the mobility and anonymity prevalent in areas of hotels and boarding-houses the fundamental causes of variations in psychosis rates within a town.

Nevertheless, ought we not to look beyond ecological factors for more powerful social or economic factors? If analysis is taken further, as it was by Belknap and Jaco, for example, who classified patients within each area according to income, marital status, religious affiliation, etc., it becomes obvious that the sociological

95

approach is needed to supplement the ecological one, and that social and ecological factors always interact. For example, Baptists, Methodists, Lutherans and Members of the Church of Christ show more mental illness than Catholics and Episcopalians living in the same area. We are therefore led from ecology to sociology in our search for the causes of personality disorders; there is no doubt about this, as Dunham himself finally admitted. We could add the following comment by Chombart de Lauwe:

> The inability of the city dweller to situate himself in physical space is not the least of the causes of the instability of our society. In the study of the relationship between the material structures of a society and its mental representations and aspirations a third element appears: social space, the image which groups and individuals form of the society they live in. An urban neighbourhood is therefore determined not only by its geography and its economy, but by the representations that its inhabitants and those of other neighbourhoods have of it.

If we apply this statement to our problem, we could say that in the aetiology of mental disorder it is necessary to take into account both the 'image' of a particular environment and its direct influence.

Psychoanalysts, who believe in the fundamental nature of the childhood trauma, accept the idea that some environments are more favourable than others, but they see them as a product of earlier and more significant causes. In their view, statistics only disguise the facts, which in reality consist of the life-histories of individuals. Thus Krout thinks that schizophrenia develops in individuals fixated at the oral stage because of frustration during feeding, while manic-depressive psychosis represents an anal fixation due to toilet training frustrations. The former type of fixation is found mainly in the poorer areas, while the latter is distributed throughout the middle-class residential areas.[23] Previously we moved from ecology to sociology, now in turn we are led to a particular area of sociology, the sociology of the family.

Nevertheless, we cannot reject *a priori* the influence of the two factors which ecologists regard as the most significant: isolation and mobility. But we must go further than a mere impressionistic view; we must review the different studies that have been made of these two phenomena, the contradictions they present and their progressive technical refinement.

3 Isolation and mobility

The first question ecologists asked—as we saw with Burgess— was whether areas of extreme social isolation play an aetiological role in certain psychoses, such as schizophrenia, or whether they merely serve as a refuge for already disturbed people. The next question that crops up is whether social isolation is a predisposing or a precipitating factor. Both questions are basically linked, because even if social isolation does not cause mental disorder, it could at least accelerate its onset, while neighbourhoods where social participation was greater would inhibit its appearance. Jaco wished to test the precise effect of this factor. He established a certain number of indices of social isolation.[24] *Anonymity.* (How many names of neighbours, friends, acquaintances can the subject give?) *Spatial mobility.* (Does the subject rent or own his home? How many times has he moved previously? How long has he been in his present home?) *Frequency of participation.* (Membership of professional, cultural, political or religious organizations.) *Rate of unemployment in the area.* And, finally, *interaction with other neighbourhoods.* (Visiting and travelling.) Using these criteria, he examined the fifteen electoral tracts of Austin, Texas, to see whether those tracts having the highest rate of schizophrenia (and manic-depressive psychosis as a control) were in fact areas where the social-isolation criteria applied. This is what he found for 668 patients studied between 1940 and 1952:

33% of the schizophrenics resided in the 9th and 10th tracts compared with 3·4% in the 1st and 15th.

29·5% of the manic-depressives resided in the 8th and 12th tracts compared with 2·6% in the 5th and 2nd.

The following factors of social isolation were found to be characteristic of high mental disorder areas:

(1) Limited contact with neighbours, friends and acquaintances.

(2) More people renting than owning their homes, but, on the other hand, apparently no more migration than in other areas.

(3) Less participation in trade-union activities and in various organizations; higher rate of electoral abstention.

(4) Greater occupational mobility.

(5) Fewer visits downtown, to friends, to other neighbourhoods, and fewer trips out of town.

Thus social isolation does have an effect, as Faris and Dunham suggested, but it is more of a precipitating factor than a predisposing one. According to Jaco, we could, broadly speaking, construct the following table:

No predisposition and social isolation: no mental disorder.
Predisposition and no social isolation: no mental disorder.

97

Both factors would be needed, the external and the internal, for disturbance to occur. Although the role of ecological factors is reduced, it is obviously still considerable.

Have we now come closer to discovering the internal factor? Faris thought childhood experience, as suggested by Krout's hypothesis, mentioned earlier, was a variable to be considered; he suggested that the child who is over-protected, particularly by his mother, will have a greater tendency than others to become schizophrenic. He subsequently rejected this idea, since the child is moulded not only by his family, but also by his school, which is an agency of socialization that may counteract the influences of the home. Therefore for the over-protected child to become a social isolate he must also be persecuted by his peers, labelled a 'sissy', made fun of and rejected. Persecution by school-mates varies according to the ecological area of the city: in well-integrated middle-class areas the affective relationship between parents and children can provide a better basis for social integration, whereas in disorganized areas—slums, melting-pot areas, and gang-lands where the criminal is idealized—the pampered child would find a barrier preventing interaction with other children of his own age in the street and in the playground. Thus, finally, ecology has the last word.[25] In fact, Faris maintains, contrary to those who think that predisposition to schizophrenia comes from childhood experience, that the life-histories of the majority of his schizophrenic subjects show a normal childhood, and that it is their isolated life in disorganized communities that much later on caused their illness.

However, Dunham found that among catatonic schizophrenics living in areas of high delinquency, many had been pampered children experiencing rejection by children from other families, failing in their efforts to make friends with their peers and gradually becoming resigned to a life of isolation.[26] Kohn and Clausen took up the question afresh. By interviewing patients and their relatives, they reconstructed the life-histories of forty-five schizophrenics in Maryland Hospital from 1940 to 1952. They used a control group of thirteen manic-depressive patients.[27] Their findings are negative: one-third of both groups of patients had been social isolates from the age of thirteen to fourteen and the others had had a normal life. No proof was found that the isolated patients were prevented from forming social relationships because of residential mobility, serious illness, or simply because of parental restriction. In the second place, the authors did not find any interrelation between social isolation and affective relations between parents and children. Predisposition, which, according to Jaco, plays such an important part aside from the external ecological factor, is to be found beyond childhood experience in the actual constitution of the subject. Social isolation is more an effect than a cause: it is an indication that the patient's difficulty in relating to others has become so great that he resigns himself to living alone. In support of their conclusions, Kohn and Clausen quote Weinberg's research on a group of schizophrenics (half of whom were catatonic) which did not show any evidence of the precipitating or predisposing effect of social isolation.[28]

We can now return to the questions we asked at the beginning of this section. All we can say at present is that the ecological area has only a precipitating effect, if any. What is more, this effect is secondary rather than primary: there tends to be a vicious circle, the person who is already psychotic chooses to live in an area of social isolation, and once in this area he is affected by it and becomes increasingly desocialized. Let us now examine the second allegedly responsible factor, spatial mobility.

Tietze, Lemkau and Cooper tried to measure the effect of this factor[29] and established two general laws: (1) There is a higher rate of mental disorder among the residentially mobile than among those who live for a long time in the same home (which would explain why there is so much more mental disorder in areas of rented accommodation than in areas of owner-occupation). The rate is higher for those who move within the same town than for those who migrate to the town from other communities. It is immediately clear that if these findings are valid they present the same sort of problem as the isolation factor. Is excessive mobility the cause of psychosis or it is psychosis which drives people to change their home continually? Is it because he is always on the move, always parting from neighbours and acquaintances, that the mobile individual has no stable social relations? Or is it to escape from his inner problems, anxieties and panic states that he moves from place to place?

The first point that needs to be emphasized is that a distinction must be made between different psychoses. In their study of ecological areas, Faris and Dunham established a correlation between residential mobility and schizophrenia. Also in Chicago, Freedman found twenty years later (perhaps because the pattern of migration had changed in that time) a very high correlation between migration and manic-depressive psychosis, whereas the correlation with schizophrenia was not significant.[30] If we juxtapose this data with Tietze's, Lemkau's and Cooper's findings mentioned above, we could formulate the following hypothesis: there is a link, the nature of which is not yet known, between manic-depressive psychosis and inter-city migration and between other disorders, particularly schizophrenia and intra-city mobility.

99

However, as we have already seen, the findings of Jaco's study of social isolation deny the effect on schizophrenia of internal mobility. Jaco found no significant difference in intra-city mobility between areas with the highest rate of schizophrenia and areas with the lowest:

High schizophrenia areas: rate of intra-city mobility, 45%
Low schizophrenia areas: rate of intra-city mobility, 55%

Lystad compared a group of schizophrenics in New Orleans with a control group of non-schizophrenic patients discharged from a private nursing home. She found that the schizophrenics were less geographically mobile than the others. However, she adds that other important differences occur when age, race and social class are taken into account: the non-schizophrenics who were middle-class, white and young and had a high level of education were more mobile than the schizophrenics in the same group; on the other hand, the non-schizophrenics who were working-class, Negro, old, and with only elementary education did not show a greater mobility than the schizophrenics in the same group.[31]

The contradictory results of the various studies reviewed do not allow us to come to any conclusions about the possible role of geographic mobility in the aetiology of psychosis. But let us note that we only mentioned (1) studies of indigenous populations. The question of foreign immigrants also needs to be considered. (2) Spatial mobility and not social mobility. We will later be faced with the question whether or not vertical mobility, i.e. mobility from one class to another, or the obstacles it encounters, play an important part in the causation of mental disturbance. But we shall then be moving out of ecological territory and into sociology.

4 Conclusions

The contribution of ecology to the sociology of mental disorder has been the discovery of definite spatial patterns in the distribution of psychoses, both organic and functional. This regular distribution cannot be due to chance, but ecology is not able to offer any definitive explanations; it can only suggest hypotheses. Broadly speaking, these hypotheses take us back a century to Auguste Comte's theory. If we retrace the history of the sociology of mental disorder, we will recall that Positivism regarded personal disorganization as a result or as a reflection of social disorganization. The only difference is that Comte studied social disorganization over time, as a characteristic of particular crisis periods in the evolution of man, while ecology is based on spatial data, and looks at social disorganization as it occurs in different environments, which can be either urban or, as we discovered, rural.

The contribution of ecology is not a bad starting-point for socio-logical research. There are ecological problem areas with concen-trations of particular psychoses, just as there are areas characterized by juvenile delinquency or sexual crimes. These areas are complex wholes where many variables, family, economic, political, religious, etc., overlap and interact with each other; ecological studies can-not control the influences of every factor. Psychosis could be the result (either primary or secondary, according to whether the en-vironment is considered to create mental disorder or merely to be a precipitant to an already disorganized personality) of all these factors added together and reinforcing each other. Or is there a main factor that eludes ecological description? As we have seen, there are certain sociologists and psychiatrists who feel that physical environment is less relevant than social class—that is, the standard of living of the population. On the other hand, some psy-chiatrists and psychoanalysts maintain that it is necessary to go back to the early experience characterstic of parent-child relations in poverty-stricken or low-income areas. Even if a high rate of psychosis in a particular area is considered to be the reflection of a whole set of factors, it may still be possible to discriminate be-tween these factors and assess their relative influence. In any case, we feel that the only factors that have interested ecologists (isolation and mobility) are not sufficiently convincing. We need to go beyond ecological descriptions to study other variables, to look at the pattern of mental disorder, not according to geographical location, but according to social class, type of family, religion, etc.

Nevertheless, from the various findings of the studies we have summarized in this chapter we can draw a few main conclusions. We had to reject the nostalgic philosophy of the first psychiatrists who considered country people were shielded from mental dis-order. This idea was linked to the Rousseauist doctrine of the first anthropologists who maintained that primitive societies were free from psychosis and particularly from schizophrenia. Their under-lying assumption was that groups that had a simple structure, a limited number of members and personal and friendly social relations were free from both intra- and inter-personal stress. Ten-sions began when social organization became more complex be-cause of an increase in population density. In reality, it is not organization that makes life difficult. There are other factors to be considered. For example, the roles offered by country life are limited and rigid; they have been crystallized by tradition and do not always correspond to the diversity of human inclinations. Certain types of individual in rural areas have to accept social roles to which they are unsuited: an enterprising young man has to behave in a submissive way towards his parents, a woman with a masculine temperament has to play a passive role, etc. On the other hand, the great variety of occupations found in the city offers a wide range of roles better adapted to the wealth of individual disposition.[32] If, according to our definition, normality consists less in following the norms of the group than in a capacity for normative activity, then who can deny that the city should be conducive to a fuller development of the personality? Organization, which is the result of population concentration, is not in itself responsible for the growth in mental illness; its rigidity and anomie are to blame. As ecological methods are improved, they were able to show that the city has its areas of alienation, but also of mental health, and the country has both healthy communities and villages where pathological processes occur.

We came to the conclusion that social isolation was not a significant factor. But this is because we saw it as characteristic of specific urban areas. In the country the isolation of certain mountain villages does have a pathological result, whereas in some closed rural communities isolation has a therapeutic and even a preventive effect. As for the city, the results of research on isolation are sometimes contradictory. But surely it is possible to rise above the restricted definitions of isolation to a broader conception that would define Western civilization in the way that the expression 'schizoid culture' does. Insularity seems to be a widespread phenomenon, not one that is limited to particular areas of social disorganization. For example, Paul Halmos was able to discover among students of two London colleges in 1948, with the use of questionnaires on social participation, the role of social isolation in the development of neurotic anxiety in the middle and upper middle classes.[33] The proof that social isolation is characteristic of our society and not only of particular groups is that it has actually become an ideology. In its Christian form it is the cultivation of the soul with a view to salvation; in its economic form it is the competition between individuals for social status, and for intellectuals, such as those studied by Halmos, it is the 'ivory tower'. What is more, in any person belonging to our civilization there is a conflict between social feelings urging him to participate and cultural norms that make him withdraw into himself. His life-style is consequently mutilated.

The defect of the studies we mentioned is not that they overestimate the importance of social isolation, but that they underestimate it by limiting it to particular geographic areas. The isolation factor needs to be 'despatialized' and related to other distributions of mental disorder. Neurosis, psychoneurosis and functional psychosis must also be taken into account. Here again we are not far removed from Comte, who defines madness as an excess of subjectivity and relates this outbreak of subjectivity to the individualistic structures of society emerging after the Reformation and the French Revolution.

V   The psychiatry of the total society: from occupation and social class to the industrial society

As we leave ecology for sociology proper, the question arises: in what order should we deal with our variables? Sociology developed parallel with industrialization; it began in France with Comte, in England with Spencer and in Germany with Marx. Its principal aim, in spite of all the additions made to it since, is still the 'natural history' of industrial society. A sociology of mental disorder would really only deserve its name if it were limited mainly to the study of the effects of industrialization and social class on mental health. However, psychiatrists, especially since Freud, are not concerned with groups, but with individuals; they try to understand the origins of mental disturbance by reconstructing the early family history of their patients with the aid of clinical material. If we wish to transfer their ideas to the framework of sociology, we must begin with the study of the family, not so much as a social institution in Durkheim's sense of the term, but as a set of interrelations between people of different sexes and ages. Because of the ambiguous nature of our discipline, which unites the two terms 'sociology' and 'mental disorder', we hesitate between these two approaches; the first is closer to the aim of sociology and the second to the aim of psychiatry. It should not be surprising that we should choose the first approach. The contemporary family is shaped by industrial society and is markedly different from the pre-industrial family. Each class has its own family type which is more or less authoritarian, democratic, paternal, maternal or egalitarian. The function of parents is to socialize children—that is, to give them the necessary mental equipment for their integration into a complex society. They must ensure that the young internalize—and that is what is known as socialization—not individual values and norms, but the values and the cultural norms of the society that surrounds them. Psychiatrists or psychoanalysts who are more sociologically oriented recognize in the end that the family is merely a bridge between society and the individual, and often only a mediator between the disturbances of industrial society and individual disturbances. Alexander, for example, maintains that the disorganization or anomie of society creates family disorganization, which in turn is reflected in individual behaviour disturbances. For example, families who are handicapped in terms of social class, income, religion, race, etc., affect the insular attitudes of their children.[1] Bossard and Boll also show that the tensions of the community as a whole are transformed into tensions within the family, which have an effect on the children.[2] Finally, Paul Halmos makes the following point:

> The socio-cultural determinants precede and control individual genetic development; the intra-familial are enclosed in the large extra-familial field, and the inner relationships of the former are fixed by the secondary institutions of the latter. Hence the process of desocialization can be understood only as a socio-cultural pathogenesis. . . . Mediation [by the family] is a mere phase of the socio-cultural process.[3]

These few examples are sufficient to justify our order of approach.

Research on the relationship between social class and psychosis is relatively recent. Perhaps the Marxists are right when they say that medical men, as members of the *bourgeoisie*, unconsciously wish to forget the crucial drama of industrial society which is the alienation of the working class (in the sociological sense, but which can also lead to mental alienation). Perhaps simply because they are psychiatrists, they are little inclined to toy with concepts far removed from their field; they are discouraged by difficulties which still puzzle sociologists today: What is social class? How many classes are there? Obviously the mentally ill can only be distributed according to social class once these classes have been defined and their number accurately established. On the other hand, their patients' files were available, brought up to date by the hospital administration, and always—or nearly always—carrying information on the patients' occupations. What is more, the growth of friendly societies organized on an occupational basis made available enough data on occupations for a fairly advanced psychosociological analysis. Thus, historically speaking, research on the pathology of various occupational groups came before research on the pathogenic effect of social-class divisions. We shall therefore start with the former. As we shall see, it leads to the wider and more serious problems of industrial society and in that respect is a good introduction to them.

105

1 The psychiatry of occupational groups

Three periods can be distinguished in the evolution of this field:

(1) The first studies were concerned with the incidence of mental illness according to occupation. Jaspers had already noted, on the basis of data reported by Romer, that professional people were those most affected by psychiatric disorders. Stern confirmed this finding and pointed out that the lowest rate of mental disorder is found among agricultural workers and the highest among professionals (dementia praecox has sometimes been called the 'sickness of professors').[4] But does each occupational group have its own particular illnesses? There are, of course, individual variations, but it is a fact that certain behaviour is often typical of a particular group, e.g. office workers, teachers or manual workers, and pathological phenomena can be determined more by the common characteristics of the group than by the individuals that constitute it. Mira's study of 6,000 clinical cases in Spanish hospitals shows drug-addiction to be predominant among intellectuals and artists, schizophrenia among philosophy and theology students, paranoid delusions among policemen, epileptic traits among domestic workers, neurasthenia among telephonists, latent homosexuality among male hairdressers, cooks, tailors and servants, and, finally, neurosis among nurses, women teachers, social workers and children's nurses (the children's nurses show evidence of latent aggression towards the mothers of children in their care). Mira gives two possible explanations for this differential pathology. In some cases a sort of preselection occurs: the psychosis develops first and the occupation is chosen precisely because it suits the pathological make-up of the person. In other cases the occupation has a direct effect on behaviour and attitudes, as with hairdressers and children's nurses: it becomes a cause of morbidity.[5] Recently there has been a profusion of monographs on particular groups or occupational settings, producing increasingly refined analyses. For example, in France we have Le Guillant's study of female domestic and agricultural workers in the light of the Marxist concept of alienation.[6] Baruk's and Guilhot's study of administrative workers examines the effects of bureaucracy and administrative practices on the mental health of individuals and groups, and the occurrence of a particular form of hypersensitiveness among employees (*psychallergie administrative*).[7] Finally, we have Berger's and Benjamin's research on teachers, which shows how the downgrading of the teaching profession in contemporary society creates feelings of frustration and psychiatric disturbances in this occupational group.[8] These various studies show that it is necessary to

consider social status in the aetiology of mental illness. We shall return to this factor later and attempt to assess its importance.

Whereas the early studies revealed that the highest incidence of mental illness was to be found among professional people, the most recent research shows that the highest rates—at least for first admissions to hospital—are found among manual workers. Thus, for the male population of Ohio, U.S.A., in 1958, agricultural workers show more schizophrenia than other occupations, and for the female population working women show more schizophrenia than housewives.[9] Frumkin compared the rate of incidence of different types of psychosis among unskilled workers and professional people: he found a greater rate of hospitalization, particularly for schizophrenia, in the first group (201·9 and 67·3 per 100,000) than in the second (22·8 and 7·2):[10]

> From his various findings, Frumkin developed the hypothesis
> that lower-class occupational groups develop mental illnesses
> which are largely sociogenic in origin, i.e. due to sociopathy,
> which is generally directed against society, while the ultra-
> conservative upper-class occupational groups have higher rates
> of mental disorders which are psychogenic in origin, i.e. due
> to psychopathy, which is generally directed against the self.
> Middle-class groups, however, suffer from both sociogenic
> and psychogenic mental disorders. Men, being more radical in
> their philosophy, are more likely to have rates which correspond
> closer to the lower-class patterns, while females, being more
> conservative, are more likely to have disorders of a psychogenic
> nature. To illustrate this, Frumkin found more manic-depressive
> psychosis, involutional melancholia and psychoneurosis, which
> are illnesses of the upper classes, among females than males. On
> the other hand, he found a greater rate of syphilis and alcoholic
> psychosis—illnesses of the lower classes—among males.[11]

We can now see that there has been a shift from the study of occupational groups to the study of social class. It looks as though we have to go beyond the occupational factor to the more crucial factor for an aetiology with a sociological orientation, the stratification of groups within the wider structure of industrial society.

At this point we are led to wonder why such a complete reversal occurred in the findings between the earlier and the later studies. It is difficult to compare results from two different periods and two different continents. It is possible that in the past intellectuals were more concerned with their mental health and tended to seek treatment more readily than other groups. It could also be that the technological revolution, with its more sudden crises, has adversely affected the lower classes. Finally, it is possible that, with the progress of sociology, statistical data have become more accurate than they were before. We can only take note of this contradiction and leave the question unanswered.

(2) The second period was marked by attempts to go beyond the data and to interpret the variations in mental disorder rates according to occupation. Two factors need to be considered in this type of analysis: salary (or income) and prestige. To separate the two factors, it would, of course, be necessary to compare occupations of different status and similar pay, or occupations of different economic level and the same social status. This is a difficult task; it partly overlaps with the problem of social class and social stratification, to be discussed later. We will therefore confine ourselves to the findings of research based on occupational categories, which originally brought this problem to light.

Clark, in 1948, interpreted the preponderance of schizophrenia in the lower occupational groups. Apart from such causes as the physical effect of certain types of work, or the importance of alcohol and sex in working-men's lives, there are three reasons for these high rates: (a) the differential attractiveness and desirability of various occupations; (b) the difference in the prestige which these jobs carry in the eyes of society; (c) the many problems created by low income and the cost of housing. Clark's study thus embraced both economic level and social status.[12] He took up the problem afresh in 1953 and, on the basis of a more comprehensive distribution of mental disorder according to occupation (see pp. 335, 340), came to the final conclusion that prestige is more important for mental health than income.[13] Frumkin, on the other hand, notes that:

(a) the highest concentrations of mental disturbance and psychosis are found in low-status occupational groups (unskilled and domestic workers), and the lowest are found among people who hold executive positions and enjoy high social status.

(b) Occupation is more important for men, because the frustrations women experience at work are compensated for by their role as wives or mothers; in fact, the social status of women is in general less determined by their own occupational status than by that of their husband. Therefore occupational prestige is more important than income for men than it is for women.[14]

Although these conclusions seem reasonable, in our opinion we should not neglect the purely economic factor. The inequality of incomes creates serious problems for workers at the bottom of the scale: some unskilled workers live in a state of permanent anxiety about the future, worrying whether they will lose their job, be refused credit by tradesmen, receive notice because they cannot pay their rent, etc. These never-ending problems can in the long run undermine mental health. It has often been noted that the reason for widespread drunkenness among lower occupational groups is that unskilled workers tend to use drink as an escape from their problems: hence their high rate of psychosis caused or complicated by alcoholism.

These studies on the significance of the income and prestige of various occupations in the aetiology of mental illness are naturally based on a scale of occupations. Here the psychiatrist needs the help of the sociologist, for a prestige scale cannot be based on subjective impressions; a preliminary survey is necessary to determine the system of collective representations underlying this scale. Sociologists can employ a number of techniques which are beyond the scope of this book, but which show that these systems vary from one culture to another. For example, in Latin America the professions, especially the legal profession, carry the most prestige, while in North America the most highly valued occupation is that of industrial executive. The rigidity and flexibility of these systems also need to be taken into account—in other words, the conditions of access to various jobs. Thus Ruesch, in connection with mental illness, contrasts European society with its more mobile North American counterpart: 'Flexibility and social change are in America the principal sources of insecurity; while in Europe social stratification and rigidity result in frustration.'[15] Here again we are led from the question of occupation to the question of social class and of the degree of rigidity or flexibility of the stratification system.

(3) Finally, parallel with the growth of industrial sociology we witness the development of industrial psychiatry, which still searches for relationships between occupation categories and behaviour disorders, but this time within the integrating framework of industry. With the development of industrial psychiatry, interest shifted from psychosis to neurosis. As many different neuroses were created as there were categories of employees in a factory, from 'executive neurosis' (the *Manager-Krankheit* of the Germans), caused by the ever-increasing strain of competition, the growing responsibilities of executives and the exhaustion which results from having to resolve conflicts within the factory so that everything runs efficiently, all the way down to the neuroses of skilled or trained workers, taking in the neuroses of clerks and accountants. The neurosis of executives usually takes a psychosomatic form: psychic disturbance is expressed in or complicated by cardiovascular syndromes. In manual workers neurosis takes many different forms, corresponding to the diversity of problems faced by the working class. For example, 'pension psychoneurosis' (G. Colin): 'the worker is hoping for a convenient accident so that he

109

can claim compensation from his employer and spend the rest of his life without working'; 'strike neurosis' (Delmas-Marsalet), 'which takes the form of obsessional delusions'; 'unemployment neurosis' (J. Vie), 'which relates in fact to popular attitudes to unemployment'. Thus Tietze, who compared the amount of mental disorder among the unemployed in Baltimore in 1933 and in 1936, found that at the latter year the number of cases was only one-third of the 1933 figure; this was because in 1936, a period of economic depression, the workers considered unemployment to be due to circumstances outside their control, a sort of inevitable catastrophe with which the Government was expected to deal.[16]

Since Mayo's classic study on the importance of workers' satisfaction for output and efficiency, industrial psychiatrists have increasingly turned their attention to the effects on productivity of neurotic conflicts. Productivity depends, of course, on the worker's professional qualities (his skills), but also on his perseverance, self-confidence and enjoyment of his work. Neurosis can endanger output by affecting these factors: (a) the worker's skills by creating in him an unconscious tendency to lower his performance rather than expose himself to ridicule; (b) his self-confidence by taking the form of self-doubt or even self-hate and an unconscious fear of failure; (c) his interest in his work, by creating imaginary and unrealistic ambitions or even a pride in not working.[17] A particularly important advance has been the recognition in the last last few decades, along with the development of occupational medicine and the general acceptance of Freudian principles in all medical fields, of the part played by unconscious conflicts in industrial accidents. It is true that figures vary from one author to another (there is an important subjective element in the assessment of the causes of an accident). The percentage of serious accidents said to be caused in this way varies between 20 per cent[18] and 80 per cent.[19] The diagnosis is mainly based on the fact that some people are accident-prone, as though they were seeking a socially acceptable form of suicide, or at least a solution to their problems by acting out their obsessions with failure; or else their accident may seem to them a revenge on society, a form of blackmail of their parents or more frequently of their wives (accidents are more frequent among married men than among young bachelors). Ever since it was recognized that work teams are conducive to productivity and that friendly relations between workers lead to higher output, interest has been growing in another problem affecting the work situation: the conflicts caused by psychologically abnormal personalities introducing themselves into a work-team and creating discord.

The whole of recent industrial psychiatry, which has progressively replaced studies of occupational categories by the study of particular neuroses affecting managers on the one hand and workers on the other, rests on two principles. The first is the utilitarian principle. This is connected with an ideology of productivity which sees internal conflicts as a serious handicap to productivity, and its logical outcome is the demand that, as well as aptitude tests, employers should use projective tests in the selection of employees, and an analyst or psychiatrist should be installed in factories. The second principle derives from the fact that most of the studies we have mentioned are the work of psychiatrists rather than sociologists, and are based more on case histories than on reflections about our society. They are therefore founded on the principle of multiplicity and variability of the neuroses, with the result that we have a conglomeration of types, each linked to a particular feature of industrialization: strikes, unemployment, the managerial revolution, etc. Clearly the sociologist would have a different approach: he would begin by studying the total structure of society in order to understand its pathology. Just as the statistics of occupational categories led us to the study of social class, industrial psychiatry brings us to the issue of contemporary society and of anomie. We will devote the next part of this chapter to these two questions.

2 Class and social stratification

It has been noted that the three main social classes which sociologists usually distinguish, the upper, middle and lower classes, do not present the same pattern of mental disorder. Thus Ruesch reports more psychosomatic conditions in the middle class, a reflection of the conformist tendencies of this class, traumatic disorders in the lower class related to the class struggle, and psychoneuroses in the upper class 'with their overbearing superego and cultural traditions'.[20] But these are statements that have to be statistically verified. Rennie and his collaborators discovered that psychosis varies in inverse relation to the scale of social stratification, and neurosis in direct relation: 13 per cent of their psychotic subjects were in the lowest class compared with 3·6 per cent in the highest; 28 per cent of the most serious cases were at the bottom of the social scale and 9 per cent at the top; finally, 25 per cent of the patients in the lowest class were neurotic compared with 43 per cent in the higher strata.[21] However, the principal work on the relation between psychiatric data and social class is the result of a close collaboration between a sociologist and a psychiatrist, Hollingshead and Redlich. Their book, which is based on data collected in New Haven, will serve as a focal point for our discussion.[22]

The two types of social stratification found in New Haven, the

111

vertical (race, ethnic group, religion) and the horizontal (residence, education, occupation), were combined to form a highly compartmentalized structure which is the sociological framework of the study. An index of social position was calculated by scoring the families according to place of residence, occupation and educational level of the breadwinner, and by giving weights to the three factors of 6, 9 and 5 respectively. On this basis the families were divided into five classes.

Class I is composed of rich families, usually inheriting their wealth, whose breadwinner tends to be an industrial executive or an administrator, whose members have received a university education, and who enjoy the highest social prestige.

Class II is composed of families living in good residential districts, also rich, but who have earned rather than inherited their wealth, and whose members have had at least secondary and often higher education.

Class III is composed of owners of small businesses, clerks and skilled manual workers, whose children sometimes reach university, but more frequently go to technical colleges, who live in good residential areas, but usually frequent different clubs or organizations from members of Classes I and II.

Table 10 Social class distribution of mental disorder

Class	Total population	Mental patients
I	3·1	1·0
II	8·1	6·7
III	46·0	13·2
IV	22·0	38·6
V	17·8	36·8
Unknown	3·0	3·7
	100·0	100·0

Class IV is composed of semi-skilled workers who—at least in the older age-groups—have only received elementary education, who live in less desirable areas and whose social life is restricted to family relationships, neighbourhood contacts and trade-union activities.

Class V, at the bottom of the scale, is composed of unskilled workers, most of whom have not even completed elementary education, who live in the most deprived areas and whose life is centred around family, street and neighbourhood.

We find that as we move down from Class I to Class V the amount of mental illness increases as shown in Table 10.

However, as Rennie pointed out, a distinction must be made between neurosis, which is predominant in the higher classes, and psychosis, which is concentrated in the lower classes. The following table confirms this pattern:

Table 11 Social class distribution of neurosis and psychosis

Class	Neurosis	Psychosis	Total
I	52·6	47·4	100·0
II	67·2	32·8	100·0
III	44·2	55·8	100·0
IV	23·1	76·9	100·0
V	8·4	91·6	100·0

Schizophrenia in particular is more frequent the lower one goes down the social scale; 0·7 per cent of the schizophrenic patients were in the upper class, and in the other four classes we find in descending order: 2·7 per cent, 9·8 per cent, 41·6 per cent and 45·2 per cent. In fact, the lowest social stratum contributes a disproportionate amount of psychotic patients, whether one considers first admissions, readmissions, acute attacks or chronic disorders:

Table 12 Incidence, readmissions and chronic cases

Class	Incidence	Re-entry	Continuous	Prevalance of Schizophrenia	Prevalance of Psychosis	Totel incidence
I & II	6	14	97	111	188	97
III	8	20	148	168	291	114
IV	10	21	269	300	518	89
V	20	46	729	895	1,505	139

Hollingshead and Redlich maintain that this regular distribution according to social class cannot be due to geographical or social mobility: 65 per cent of the New Haven schizophrenics had been living in the same area for many years, and only 35 per cent were migrants. The authors collected life histories for the patients in Class V to test whether, according to Burgess's theory, these patients had deliberately taken refuge in zones of social disorganization, or whether, as Faris and Dunham suggest, the environment produces the psychosis. These life histories revealed that the patients had always lived in the same area. The effect of social mobility must also be ruled out, as the great majority of the patients were non-mobile:

Table 13 Vertical mobility and mental disorder

Vertical Mobility	Classes I & II	Class III	Class IV	Class V
Patient and family not mobile	20	54	322	345
Patient upward from family	7	19	6	—
Patient downward from family	1	2	3	4
Insufficient data	1	8	21	39
	29	83	352	383

In other words, 91 per cent of the patients were not mobile compared with 1·3 per cent who were in a lower class and 4·4 per cent who were in a higher class.

The conclusion which emerges from this data (although the authors subsequently replied to their critics that they had not intended to make an aetiological study) is that the crucial factor in determining the total incidence of mental disorder and the ratio of psychosis to neurosis is social stratification. 'Lower-class living seems to stimulate the development of psychotic disorders. We infer from our data that the excess of psychoses from the poorer area is a product of the life conditions entailed in the lower socio-economic strata of society' (p. 242). Hollingshead and Redlich did not limit themselves to this aetiological analysis: they also showed the influence of economic status on therapy. This question was dealt with by Myers and Schaeffer, who found that patients of high social status were accepted for psychotherapy more readily, were treated by a more highly qualified therapist and stayed in hospital longer.[23] Hollingshead and Redlich's table shows the close relationship between type of treatment and social class:

Table 14 Social class and type of therapy

Class	Psychotherapy	Organic therapy	Custodial care, no treatment	Total
I	73·7	10·5	15·8	100·0
II	81·7	11·4	6·9	100·0
III	52·7	28·7	18·6	100·0
IV	31·3	37·1	31·8	100·0
V	16·1	32·7	51·2	100·0

These particular facts are beyond question, even in our democratic society. But we must point out that the aetiological findings of Hollingshead and Redlich for New Haven are not borne out by authors who have studied other communities. Graham, for example, in his Pennsylvania study, found more serious psychiatric disturbance, at least of an acute type, in the higher than in the lower classes.[24] In Ontario Laughton found no significant differences between upper, middle and lower classes for all illnesses, for psychiatric disturbances and for psychosomatic disorders.[25] An even more striking fact is that, contrary to what is maintained by Hollingshead and Redlich and a great many European and American psychiatrists, Lemkau, Tietze and Cooper's study of the Baltimore district showed that neurosis was not concentrated in the upper class, but, like psychosis, was relatively more frequent in the lower classes.[26] We cannot ignore these contradictions. They cast doubts on the findings reported in *Social Class and Mental Illness*. We must therefore submit these findings to critical examination before we can accept them.

This criticism can be divided into two parts: criticism of methodology and criticism of interpretation.

Kaplan questioned the validity of statistics based on hospitalization figures. He pointed out that patients from higher socioeconomic backgrounds have a much greater likelihood of being nursed at home or of receiving treatment in private nursing homes than lower-class patients, who have no choice but to enter public mental hospitals. This explains why the figures show so much more mental illness in the underprivileged classes; hospitalized psychotics do not give a true indication of the social-class distribution of mental disorder.[27] Hollingshead and Redlich did try to provide a complete picture for New Haven, but they admitted that they were not successful. Two Connecticut psychiatrists refused to make their files available, and their patients, who were from the higher ranks of the community, were therefore not included in the statistical analysis. Nineteen New York psychiatrists were reluctant to co-operate; they had thirty patients between them, again in the highest class. Finally, seventy-two cases were omitted from the final figures because of insufficient clinical or sociological data, or because only their diagnostic category was known (they were classified according to probability calculated from the diagnostic breakdown of the 1,895 cases on whom data were available). Fifty of these omitted cases are from the highest class; when they are added to the 150 of Classes I and II, we obtain a total non-response rate of 10 per cent, close to the total population of these two groups (11·4).[28] The pattern is then very different, and the higher classes do not appear to be as favoured by their circumstances as they first appeared.

As for the interpretation of the data, we must first point out that Hollingshead and Redlich did not discover any correlation between social class and mental disturbance, whether for men or women, in the 15 to 24 years age-group. This fact is certainly curious: it limits the social-class interpretation, at least for a particular sector of the population. Secondly, they found a link between family disorganization and personal disorganization:

Table 15 Family disorganization and psychic disorganization

Class	Ratio of widowed to divorced or separated persons	% of broken homes	Prevalence of schizophrenia	Prevelance of Psychosis
I	27 to 1	3·4	111	188
II	9 to 1	5	—	—
III	6 to 1	10	168	291
IV	2 to 1	18	300	518
V	0·7 to 1	41	895	1,505

We may therefore wonder which is the most important explanatory factor, social status or the disorganization of the family. Family disorganization does vary markedly according to social class, but this new interpretation implies that social class operates not directly, but through the intermediary of the family.

A psychoanalytic approach would take things much further than this; the importance of social class is recognized, but the question is whether it operates, not as an element of the social structure, but in terms of differential child-rearing practices, the degree of parental strictness, or the type of frustrations imposed on the child (oral or anal). We shall return to this subject at length when we look at family factors in mental illness. Let us just mention in this context that this is the approach taken by Warner, Green, and Roberts and Myers in explaining why and how membership of a particular social class can affect the psychopathology of the individual.[29]

Aside from child-rearing, there is an equally important factor suggested by Warner: social mobility. Hollingshead and Redlich, as we have seen, rejected this factor, under the pretext that mental disorders are found more frequently among non-mobile families. But this is precisely where the problem lies. In a society like ours, where competitiveness and the ambition to improve one's status are so highly valued, social mobility is an ideal; the working class, especially the unskilled workers, find that because of their circumstances they cannot live up to the ideal of mobility, and the result is a particularly pathogenic type of frustration. It is therefore not surprising to find more psychosis or neurosis in families who cannot change their status than in those who are upwardly mobile. So we must not see social stratification as a static phenomenon where the individual's position on the social scale is the only important factor; it is a dynamic process with its bottle-necks, dead-ends and short-cuts. Hollingshead, Ellis and Kirby tried to measure the effect of the mobility factor, using a control group for the New Haven sample. They concluded that while mobility is not the only factor nor even the principal one, it is still of importance in relation to schizophrenia and psychoneurosis: social pressures create a generalized anxiety which encourages mobility and at the same time the fear of failure.[30] Mary Lystad, who compared two groups of the same class, race, sex, and educational level in New Orleans, found that the mobility of the schizophrenic group was consistently lower than that of the controls. This led her to the same conclusion that schizophrenia is concentrated in the sector of the population that wishes to rise, but that cannot achieve the desired status.[31] The results of research done in England are similar. Morrisson found that there was a definite tendency for schizophrenics to belong to a lower social stratum than their parents, especially in Class V; 48 per cent of the patients in this sample belonged to this class, while only 18 per cent of their parents did.[32] Thus it is possible that the important factor is not social class, but the increasing rigidity of a class system, which obstructs upward mobility and no longer allows the free access from one class to another which was characteristic of the early stages of capitalism. If Hollingshead's and Redlich's findings are valid, this factor may indeed be responsible for the higher frequency of disturbance in the lower strata.

3   The psychiatry of industrial society

The ecological model of concentric zones has been tentatively applied to all social problems, from divorce and juvenile delinquency to mental illness, as if a single law of spatial distribution was, or could be, proven, i.e. the progressive decrease of pathological phenomena from the centre to the periphery. The concentrations of personal disintegration (mental disorder) correspond to the concentrations of family disintegration (desertion, broken homes), and of social disintegration (crime). Does sociology also have a model which can be applied to pathological phenomena in general, and which would enable us to introduce the temporal dimension into social structures?

It would seem that Durkheim, in *The Division of Labour in Society*, has actually provided this framework when he distinguishes four types of solidarity: mechanical solidarity, organic solidarity, enforced solidarity (characteristic of colonial and slave-owning societies) and anomie. Durkheim had the merit of trying out his sociological framework himself in *Suicide*, where he applied it to a particular pathological phenomenon. He showed that the two first types of solidarity, the mechanical and the organic, correspond to two types of suicide, altruistic suicide and egotistic suicide. Enforced solidarity and anomie correspond to an abnormal increase in the suicide rate: in the society of enforced solidarity the slave kills himself to escape from bondage; anomie, which creates heightened anxiety, unbridled ambitions, vast and unrealistic plans, and at the same time makes failure more likely, is particularly conducive to suicide. A few years later, in one of the first issues of the journal founded by Durkheim, *L'Année Sociologique*, Gaston Richard attempted to show that criminality also was related to the nature of solidarity. The mechanical solidarity found under the Russian Tsarist régime produces infractions of a political and religious nature—in other words, a criminality directed against collective beliefs and the values and feelings of the community. The mechanical solidarity typical of industrialized Anglo-Saxon countries is characterized by fraud and crimes against property. Colonial solidarity, which is found in Central and South America, is characterized by sexual crimes, crimes against the person, assassinations and assault. As for the anomie of urban societies, it is conducive, through gangs, organized crime and 'underworld culture', to every sort of delinquency. Finally, Richard described the particularly violent type of criminality traditional in Mediterranean countries, such as Spain, Corsica and southern Italy, where there is a weakening of the power of the State: the political authorities are incapable of enforcing the law, with the result that the injured party takes his own revenge. However, as the State regains its power, as in Corsica, or the society becomes industrialized, as in northern Italy, criminality evolves towards the industrial type (crimes against property). Among the proofs Richard gives of the aetiological effect of these different forms of solidarity, we will retain only one: a single sociological event, such as an economic crisis, can have different manifestations according to whether the solidarity is mechanical or organic: thus in Russia it produces vagrancy and mendicancy, and in industrialized Germany a recrudescence of crimes against property.[33]

It seems that family pathology also can be interpreted meaningfully on the basis of these ideal types of solidarity. It has been found that desertion predominates in traditional Catholic peasant societies (socially rather than spiritually Catholic)—that is, in societies of mechanical solidarity; divorce in urban industrial Protestant societies, or organic solidarity societies; and polygamy, both simultaneous and consecutive (in the form of concubinage), in the old colonial and multi-racial societies; finally, anomie is reflected in the crisis of the modern family.

We may now wonder whether Durkheim's framework should not serve as a basis for a genuine sociology of mental disorder. Unfortunately, the data on mental disorder are less reliable and have much less continuity than the data on suicide or crime. They are particularly patchy for primitive societies of mechanical solidarity, the object of so much controversy among ethnopsychiatrists. However, let us try to trace hypothetically the main lines of this 'sociology of insanity'. As far as mechanical solidarity is concerned, we cannot assert that small primitive societies and folk societies are immune from mental illness, nor that they are totally unacquainted with at least the simple forms of schizophrenia.[34] However, all the studies made seem to prove that their personality disorders take on a religious character: madness is a manifestation of the divine. We therefore find in these societies the same characteristics for mental illness as for suicide (altruistic) and for crime (against collective values). In modern societies of organic solidarity we find—as with suicide and crime—'egotistic' and 'individualistic' forms of mental illness, an excessive subjectivity which escapes all social and cultural control, and an impairment of interpersonal communication. As for the enforced solidarity of Latin American countries, it is reflected in the dichotomy between the psychopathology of the white population (constitutional psychosis) and of the indigenous population or the population of African origin (organic psychosis), a state corresponding to the master-slave or master-serf duality.[35] Finally, anomie, the unregulated competition between social classes, has been the subject of numerous studies by American psychiatrists, as we have shown in our previous section.

These few remarks suggest that Durkheim's theory could well provide a framework for the sociology of mental disorder. The reason we have not used it as a basis for our analysis is that we do not have enough reliable statistical information to test the hypothesis we have suggested. In fact, we only begin to get workable sets of data with the advent of industrialization—that is, for only two forms of solidarity out of four, organic solidarity and anomie. We will therefore limit ourselves in this chapter to outlining a psychiatry of industrial society.[36]

But before we start we must take note of two things. First of all, we must consider, besides the specifically social dimensions, the cultural dimension. Industrial society cannot be understood without constant reference to the values, collective ideals and cultural norms of this society. For example, the prime value placed on individual effort and on initiative, and the ideals of productivity and upward social mobility, mediated by a whole system of norms and behaviour, put pressure on the individual and shape his attitudes. Karen Horney, to quote only one author, shows, in relation to the 'neurosis of our time', the link between neurosis and the ideals and norms of competitive capitalism:

> Among the factors in Western civilization which engender potential hostility, the fact that this culture is built on individual competitiveness probably ranks first. The economic principle of competition affects human relationships by causing one individual to fight another, by enticing one person to surpass another, and by making the advantage of one the disadvantage of the other. As we know, competitiveness not only dominates our relations in occupational groups, but also pervades our social relations, our friendships, our sexual relations and the relations within the family group, thus carrying the germs of destructive rivalry, disparagement, suspicion and begrudging envy into every human relationship.[37]

But competitive capitalism is only one form of capitalism. The next dimension we have to consider is the historical one. During the early formative period of capitalism, the religious mentality gave way to the practical mentality (Max Weber), a process which is known today as 'secularization'; this was the period during which industry grew out of such pre-industrial institutions as the artisan class and patrimonialism. After this there was a period of liberal capitalism which dominated the whole of the nineteenth century and was founded first on competition, then on the formation of trusts and cartels to avoid the disastrous effects of competition on the industrialist class. These monopolies must be considered part of liberal capitalism, since such powerful associations could only come into being through the ruthless elimination of the weaker firms. The twentieth century saw the advent of the 'second Industrial Revolution', with the appearance of a new source of power, nuclear energy, and the progress of production techniques, from the assembly line to full automation. If we wanted to summarize briefly the features of the new industrial society, we should say that it is marked by increasing organization, greater bureaucracy in firms and a division between ownership and management; as a result of economic crises, increasing State intervention in industry, even in the privately owned sector, economic planning geared to the needs of the masses and, finally, the growing importance of financial and labour pressure-groups represented by the large banks and the trade unions. During the last two decades in particular a new phase of industrialization has spread from the United States to Europe: the industrialization of agriculture.

A sociological study of mental disorder cannot neglect this historical dimension. For example, Erich Fromm, in one of his best-known books, *The Fear of Freedom*, describes the period when industrial society emerged from the ruins of feudal society. He showed that the disappearance of the security given to the working class by the guild system was not compensated for by the opportunities for personal success offered by small family enterprises and the first factories—granted that the worker could rise and could even become an employer. But he could also sink: from being a free artisan he could end up a mere labourer with only his man-power to sell. This is why the period was marked by a crisis in mental health which can be understood, not by a structural analysis of the psychiatric disorders of the time, since the data are missing, but indirectly, by analysing the compensatory ideologies of the period, such as those of the Protestant Reformation. A second example of the importance of the historical dimension is the contradiction we detected between the findings of Hollingshead and Redlich, and those, for example, of Graham. It might be possible to assume, as some psychiatrists have done, that if psychosis and neurosis are no longer predominant in the lower social strata, this is because the conditions of the working class, under the protection of the trade unions, are improving every day; earnings are increasing, and in particular they are becoming more regular. The contradiction between the two sets of data would then disappear, since they would merely be reflecting two different periods in the history of industrial society.

A striking aspect of contemporary industrial civilization is that, after being confined for a long time to Western countries, it is now progressively invading the entire world. Of course, the industrialization of under-developed countries is not really comparable to what took place in Europe from the eighteenth century onwards. In the latter case the phenomenon was endogenous, but in rural countries today it is of exogenous origin; it consequently skips stages, speeds up processes, and is infinitely more dangerous to mental health. Whole societies have to make a leap, with hardly any transition period, from the pre-capitalist to the capitalist mentality, from a cyclical to a linear conception of time, from tradition to a Promethean sacrilege. The modern factory creates the city, and the city in turn sucks in the population; it attracts rural workers who become de-tribalized; it tries to impose new norms on them and disrupts the extended family, which is reduced to a nuclear family. Asia, Africa and other parts of the world have become like building-lots where much demolition is taking place and very little building. It is difficult to evaluate the cost of the operation: Margaret Mead was asked by UNESCO to draw up a report on the state of the Third World.[38] It is true that urbanization has more effect on neurosis than on psychosis: traditional cultures also have their pathology.[39] It is also true that when acculturation takes place at a slower pace, 'cultural alternatives' provide a possibility for the basic personality to adapt itself to change.[40] But there is no doubt that, especially since decolonization, many different anxiety-provoking situations have arisen: the new industrial or administrative executives live in fear of losing their jobs through incompetence; men become afraid of losing their authority over their children and womenfolk; migrants from the country find themselves isolated in towns; people fail in their attempt to learn a new way of life. Consequently, anxiety neuroses have grown in number and severity, and the frequency of atypical schizophrenic reactions, such as delusions of persecution, are on the increase. Carothers calculated that for the whole of Africa there are 2·3 cases of mental disorder per 100,000 population in traditional areas, but that this rate increases to 13·3 for urbanized Africans.[41]

This pathology of 'transition', as it is called by Lambo, one of those who know the situation best from the inside, is also present in Western countries: industrial society is in a perpetual state of transition. The factor which is harmful to the individual in this process of change, as Leighton remarks, is not the pace at which evolution takes place, but its irregularity. The different sectors of society—or within the same sector, what Gurvitch calls the different levels of social reality—do not all evolve at the same speed. We live in a multi-temporal world and it is the discrepancy between different levels, the clash between temporalities, which, according to many psychiatrists, are responsible for the 'neurosis of our time'. Karen Horney showed how the individual learns in the family the traditional Christian values of devotion to others, self-sacrifice and altruism, only to be thrown into a competitive world, where he is expected to be aggressive and to think only of himself. There is a 'cultural lag' between family values and economic values which is expressed by a painful inner conflict, guilt-feelings and a permanent climate of anxiety.[42] Another source of anxiety is the increasingly rapid progress, not only of production techniques and mechanization, but of rationalization techniques: the quality which is increasingly required of both manager and worker is the ability to adjust to change, adaptability; the manual worker needs to be able to move from place to place and from job to job, he has to be able to change his motions continually and learn new skills; the executive has to plan for an uncertain future—he must take decisions based on long-range predictions which may later prove wrong. Hence the nervous and psychic exhaustion of present-day man. 'Fear may not slow down pioneers and heroes, but fatigue and anxiety deaden the ordinary man.'[43] And there are more ordinary men in the world than heroes.

Manual work has become either more and more fragmented and devoid of satisfaction for the worker or increasingly mechanical: automation may well do away with muscular fatigue, but it replaces it with nervous fatigue. Work, which once was considered conducive to mental well-being (to the extent that psychiatrists created occupational therapy to give patients the benefit of this mental discipline), is today, on the contrary, becoming destructive of mental health. In an excellent report presented at a French Language Conference on Psychiatry and Neurology, Y. Pélicier says the following:

> There is an increasingly clear-cut division between tasks involving control and responsibility, and those confined to repetitive activities. The first produce intellectual and emotional strain in executives, managers, engineers and technicians, which is reflected in a proliferation of minor psychic disturbances and psychosomatic ailments. The most telling illustration is what might be called the 'syndrome of the newly-promoted': the individual feels overpowered by the task he has to accomplish and looks back longingly to his previously obscure and reassuring job.
>
> In a more general way the change in the nature of work since the introduction of mechanization and automation appears to produce a reduction in physical fatigue and an increase in psychological stress. Although work has become less unpleasant in general, the pace at which some people have to work, the inhuman time-tables to which they must conform, produce many cases of anxiety and adjustment problems.[44]

At the same time, owing to technical progress, leisure is becoming more and more important in working-class life. It could serve as a safety-valve to counteract the alienating effect of occupations which have become joyless and absurd. But contemporary man cannot find fulfilment in leisure any more than in work, for the mass media only tend to replace one form of stultification by another, which is, if anything, more inhuman than the first.[45]

Another particularly pathogenic feature of industrial society is that production is geared only to profit. The needs of the consumer must be increased and new ambitions and cravings must continually be stimulated. We do not deny the good side of the affluent society. People are no longer content with just living; they want to live as well as possible. But at some point a gap occurs between the ever-growing needs and the means of satisfying them. The dream always exceeds the realities of life represented by the wage-packet, the amount of overtime available and the feasibility of a second job during the leisure-time left by the first; general affluence multiplies the sources of frustration. Kluckhohn condemns the American way of life in these words: 'It has provided the constant overstimulation necessary to throw many of us into a perpetual state of neurotic indecision.'[46] Read Bain sees in the contradiction between the build-up of needs by advertising and the impossibility of satisfying them the source of a whole series of pathological phenomena from masochism and paranoia to regressive symptoms and escape into phantasy.[47]

Pre-war psychiatry stressed the importance of the rural exodus and the difficulties of adjustment experienced by country people leaving a thriving and organic *milieu* for an artificial and sterile one. But today the instability of industrial society takes the form of a continuous movement of populations unable to grow roots anywhere or to develop in a harmonious way. The 1960 Census in the United States showed that between 1955 and 1960 around 30 million people (18 per cent of the population over five) moved from one state to another, and 13 million moved within county boundaries. Although mobility is not so great in France, it is still an important phenomenon. The rate of psychiatric disorder in Paris is higher among provincial people than among Parisian natives; those suffering most from their transplantation tend to come from the western *départements*, Alsace and central France.[48] Housing projects are never able to keep pace with the flow of people to urban centres and can only provide inadequate solutions (as we have seen in the case of high-density housing estates). Squatter communities are typical of the outskirts of towns in developing countries; their effect on mental health has been studied by psychiatrists—in Peru, for example. Overcrowded living conditions, whether in the old form of slums or in the modern form of low-cost public housing, create a typical form of neurosis (*névrose des mal-logés*), which was the subject of a thesis by Y. Girard.[49] In predisposed subjects it can even develop into persecution mania:

> Physical promiscuity and the lack of sound-proofing which contains in itself the seeds of mental automatism, create a feeling of being intruded on by others: other people become the omnipresent enemy. Members of the family are no longer in a privileged position, since spatial conditions place them on the same footing as neighbours; they are consequently also seen as intruders and become the object of the same hostility and rejection.[50]

State planning is a feature of contemporary industrial society. It can take different forms, as Gurvitch pointed out; indicative planning in fully organized capitalist societies, techno-bureaucratic control in fascist societies, communist State planning and pluralistic collectivism.[51] How do these different structures compare from the point of view of mental disorder? It is difficult to answer this question, since truly reliable data are lacking. We can only be impressionistic. At any rate, the fact that social psychiatry has recently been introduced into the Yugoslav university programme proves that social psychiatry has a place even under a system of pluralistic planning, whereas theoretically this is the sort of system which should be the least affected by psychiatric problems. In Russia statistics are based on ideological assumptions. Psychoses considered to be of organic origin are recognized, but their number is expected to remain constant. As for the neuroses, the communists consider that they have disappeared, since the end of the class struggle has eliminated the stresses of the capitalist system. But have they really disappeared? According to Western psychiatrists who have visited the U.S.S.R. they have merely been converted into psychosomatic disturbances: they are therefore treated in general hospitals along with purely somatic ailments. The propaganda systems of such régimes as fascism or communism mask the facts of mental pathology and prevent further investigation in a field which could be of great instructive value to our own planners.

Up to now we have only mentioned the most significant features of the psychiatry of industrial society. There are others, but we can only refer the reader to the more general picture of the morbidity of present-day society given in Pélicier's book, which we mentioned earlier. Pélicier's approach is more relevant to social psychopathology or to social pathology than to psychiatry proper.

What conclusions can we draw from this collection of facts?

(1) We made a distinction at the beginning of this book between morbidity rates and hospitalization rates: we pointed out that to a large extent the increase in the number of hospital patients is due to the greater availability of facilities for the treatment of cases that previously would not have come to anyone's attention. We can now add a few qualifications to this statement. It is important to note that morbidity rates have only been investigated recently and in relation to our industrial society. We cannot therefore use them as a basis for the statement that there has been no increase in mental disturbance with the progression from mechanical to organic solidarity, or from pre-industrial to industrial society. The number of 'predisposed' people may have remained more or less constant, but whereas they used to be protected by society, so that disturbance and perhaps more particularly severe disturbance were never allowed to break out, these people are now at much greater risk.

Modern civilization presents such a multitude of problems and life is becoming so difficult that solutions can no longer be found: those who used to survive, albeit by maintaining a precarious equilibrium, are now plunged into the abyss of mental illness. Duchêne notes that between 1900 and 1942, while the rate of organic psychosis remained more or less constant, the rate of reactive psychosis shot up, as though people were compelled more and more to use mental illness as a means of expressing their reactions of pain or defence, faced with a social situation which allows them no other outlet than 'madness'.[52]

(2) Because of their preoccupation with the problems of industrial psychiatry, psychiatrists have tended to confine themselves to the field of neurosis. This preference could be interpreted by the fact that neurosis is easier to analyse, while the causes of psychosis are more mysterious and difficult to unearth. One may in fact wonder whether neurosis and psychosis ought to be regarded as empirical nosological entities or whether they are not in fact 'ideal types' in the Weberian sense—the extremities of a scale between which lies a whole continuum of observable disorders. This would seem to be the orientation of the contemporary school of dynamic psychiatry, with its concept of neurosis evolving towards psychosis or near-psychosis. However, it is not up to the sociologist to settle this psychiatric issue. All we can say is that if contemporary industrial society is pathogenic, then its pathogenic effect is related, in the eyes of the psychiatrist, more to an increase in neurosis than in psychosis.

VI   The psychiatry of social groups: I. Religious groups

The individual is an integral part of society and culture, a cog in the total machine, but because of the division of labour he only plays a few of an almost unlimited number of social roles, and his participation in society as a whole is limited to a few of its sectors. One may ask whether he is not more deeply influenced by the groups to which he belongs than by the community at large; whether his mental health or ill-health are not more related to this direct influence than to the more diffuse influence of the whole on its component elements. In any case, both in individual case studies and in statistical research, problems of design and especially of control are much easier when research is restricted to particular sectors and does not try to cover an entire population or an entire culture. The present chapter and the next two will be devoted to the research that has been done on the psychiatry of social groups.

At the end of the previous chapter we roughly constructed a psychiatric sociology, using a Durkheimian framework. Now, Durkheim showed that religion is an integrative force, and he found that suicide varied in inverse relation to the integrative character of the religion. There were more suicides among Protestants than among Catholics, among Catholics than Jews, as though the individual, by putting himself under the wing of a collectivity-oriented church, became freed from his obsession with his problems; as though suicide were directly related to the individualism and lack of community spirit of the religion. Could the same be said for mental disorder? Dayton found that the rate of mental illness, exactly like the suicide rate, was higher among Protestants than Catholics and among Catholics than Jews.[1] This is a concrete example of the contrast we encountered before between two types of pathology: the first is characteristic of mechanical solidarity and the second of organic solidarity. It is true that other authors, such as Stonequist, for example, maintain on the contrary that Jews are more vulnerable to mental disorder than members of other religions.[2] However, the Jews are more than a religious group; they are also an ethnic group; as a religious group they may in fact (for reasons which Durkheim gives) be psychologically better protected, but as an ethnic group that has been persecuted in the past and still often suffers today from discrimination and oppression they are liable to undergo psychic stress detrimental to mental health. Klineberg's statistics for New York State show that in 1917 the Jews represented 16 per cent of the population of the state, but only 11·6 per cent of hospitalized mental patients were Jewish. In New York City the percentages were respectively 25·8 per cent and 16·5 per cent (the latter figure even dropping to 14·5 in 1918). On the other hand, the Jews showed at the same period the highest rate of psychoneurosis in the U.S.A.: 25·2 per cent, compared with 17 per cent for native Americans.[3] This contrast between psychosis and neurosis expresses clearly in our opinion the dichotomy between religious and ethnic membership. It reflects the difference between an integrated group of interdependent people, with its community spirit and lively religious culture, and a persecuted and rejected group whose members' clumsy attempts to sever themselves from their own people and to become assimilated into the dominant value-system are faced with an insuperable barrier.

We may therefore accept Durkheim's hypothesis on the sociological role of religion as our point of departure. But what do we mean by 'religion'? Do we simply mean the statistical fact of belonging to a group without necessarily accepting its faith, which merely denotes a person's origin and the fact of his having been baptized? Or should the word be taken, in its fullest sense, to mean a deep mystical experience? Surely it is only in the second sense that religion has an integrative value, whereas it has no effect on those who are only nominal Christians and do not take part in the life of the Church. This is the opinion of Oates, for example, who feels that it is the individual's religious experience that has to be considered, not his affiliation to a Church. However, it would be true to say that free-thinking Catholics, Protestants or Jews have grown up in an environment which, even if it is non-practising, has nevertheless retained the particular values, whether collectivity-oriented or individualistic, of the traditional faith; it is also true that child-rearing practices vary according to religious background. In France there are many examples of atheists who behave like Catholics and live according to the values inherited from their ancestors; they have merely secularized the Christian ideals without really changing their way of thinking.[4] The psychiatrist needs to take the individual's religious culture into account as well as his religious experience.

We shall therefore examine successively these two aspects of religion, first as a group to which the individual belongs, without considering whether he applies his religious principles to his everyday life, and then as a set of personal experiences shaped by dogmas which the individual believes in and practices to which he faithfully adheres.

1 Mental disorder and religious affiliation

There are two sources of data available on the Jewish religion: the present state of Israel and the Jews of the Diaspora.

In 1931 a survey of mental disorder in Israel showed a higher rate of illness among Jews than among non-Jews: 211 per 100,000 Jewish adults compared with 167 for Christians and 112 for Muslims; among the Jews there were more mentally-ill women than men. In 1936 Halpern studied 726 cases in psychiatric and neurological hospitals and confirmed the predominance of women over men. He also found that the prevalence of different types of psychosis varied according to religion.[5]

Table 16 Mental disorder and religion in Israel

	Jews	Christians	Muslims
Endogenous psychosis	81·7	68·1	71·1
Alcoholic or syphilitic psychosis	1·2	6·8	10·1
Other	17·1	25·1	18·8
	100·0	100·0	100·0

More recently Halévi found an improvement in mental health: the rate of first admissions to hospital has fallen to 140 per 100,000 population. There are more cases of manic-depressive psychosis among women and more schizophrenia and psychopathy among men. But Halévi considered in particular the two following factors: (1) The possible effect of migration to a new country. Since immigrants to Israel come from every part of the world, the mental disorders they exhibit can reflect the pattern of their country of origin.[6] This was already noted by Hes in 1958. In his sample of 124 mentally-ill immigrants from Europe, there were 11 cases of hypochondria, of whom 4 were schizophrenic, but among 124 Oriental immigrants, 40 were hypochondriac and 24 of these were schizophrenic. The only explanation in Hes's opinion is that Oriental culture tends to be more aware of hypochondria than Western culture.[7] The mental-illness pattern can also reflect problems of adjustment, especially for Oriental Jews transplanted to a modern Westernized country.[8] Thus psychosis tends to predominate among the older immigrants who arrived before the creation of the State of Israel and neurosis among the Jews who arrived during the period of mass immigration, while both forms of disorder are minimal among native Israelis.

(2) The possible influence of ecological and community factors.[9] This is reflected in the fact that the highest rate of mental disorder is found in immigrant villages where the population is not yet settled, and the lowest rate in agricultural co-operatives with a strong community spirit. (The apparent exception of the *kibbutzim* can be explained, according to the author, by their members' high cultural level and consequent greater recourse to medical treatment.[10]) This is an example of assimilative function of the religious group in a 'secularized' form.

This brief survey was necessary in order to make a comparison with the Jews of the Diaspora. For Jews in England and Wales the clinical picture is not very different from Israel (psychosis rate, 67 per 100,000 population compared with 67·2 for Israel; neurosis rate, 17 compared with 15·6 for Israel). Klineberg's figures for New York State, which we gave earlier, showed a higher rate of neurosis for the Jews of the Diaspora than for the Israeli Jews. But the high rate of neurosis among Jews could simply be due to the fact that when they are troubled by problems they tend to consult a psychiatrist more readily than members of other religions. Srole and his collaborators found that 40 per cent of patients consulting psychiatrists were Jewish, 22·7 per cent Protestant and 11·2 per cent Catholic.[11] Similarly, Hollingshead and Redlich found that in New Haven Jewish people tend to seek treatment more often than any other group.[12] Another important fact is that this concern about mental health is shared by both middle- and lower-class Jews. So we should not be misled by the difference between first-admission figures for the Israelis and the Jews of the Diaspora, especially since a study by Sanua (to be discussed later) showed that in the delusions of Jewish schizophrenics it was very exceptional indeed to find any references to persecution by the community around them. It is necessary, if we wish to discover the significance of religious affiliation, to make sure of controlling all the possible variables.

As we mentioned at the beginning of this chapter, methods of training children vary according to the religious background and traditions of the family. This variable is an important one in the aetiology of schizophrenia: it has often been suggested that the domineering mother and the passive father are typical of the families of schizophrenics. To give only one example, Barrabee and Van Mering studied sixty-nine Protestant, Catholic and Jewish psychotics in Boston. They came to the conclusion that the Jewish mother is more over-protective than the Protestant mother; the Jewish father tends to leave the responsibility for the children's upbringing to his wife, while in the Protestant family the parents tend to compete in showing affection to their children.[13] But although the authors controlled the family variable, they did not control social class, which is clearly an important factor in determining differences in child-rearing.

Myers and Roberts did control this variable. They took a sample of fifty cases, including Catholics of foreign origin and Anglo-Saxon Protestants and Jews belonging to two classes (Hollingshead and Redlich's classes III and V). It appeared that the general living conditions of the social class—for example, the disorganization of the family in Class V—were responsible for the psychopathological features. The religion variable was no longer of any significance.[14]

The great merit of Sanua's study is that it tries to control all the variables, type of family, economic status, sex and ethnic group—his Catholics belonged to both Irish and Italian immigrant groups—in relation to the various types of schizophrenia. This enables him to discover which factors are really related to religious affiliation.[15] Table 17 shows the distribution of the schizophrenics he studied.

From the socioeconomic point of view, it appears that Protestants are more mobile than Jews, but that schizophrenia is not related to upward or downward mobility. Jewish parents do prove ambitious for their children and anxious that they should succeed, but whether failure is the cause of illness or whether it is illness that produces failure is a question we cannot answer without a control group of normal Jews and Protestants. As for familial relations, the Jewish father seems more submissive and the mother more unstable; the Protestant mother is as over-protective as the Jewish mother, but the father is stricter. This depends, of course, on the type of schizophrenia (there is more parental rejection in cases of paranoid than of catatonic schizophrenia), on the social class and on the religion (the percentages of rejection and over-protection are similar for middle- and lower-class Jews, but there is more rejection

Table 17 Type of schizophrenia, social class and religious affiliation

Type	Men		Women
	Lower class	Middle class	Lower class
Jews:			
Paranoid	69	13	25
Catatonic	71	12	33
Hebephrenic	29	—	—
Protestants:			
Paranoid	60	30	—
Catatonic	21	10	28
Hebephrenic	24	—	31
Irish:			
Paranoid	34	—	—
Catatonic	16	—	—
Hebephrenic	20	—	—
Italians:			
Paranoid	26	—	—
Catatonic	20	—	—
Hebephrenic	17	—	—

among middle-class Protestants (70 per cent) than among lower-class Protestants (38 per cent)). For Catholics parental relations also depend on another variable, the ethnic group: there is much more over-protection on the part of Italian parents and more rejection in

133

Irish families. So if the family does play a role, it is only in the context of the Jewish culture, the Protestant culture or the Catholic culture. The different variables only operate in relation to the general characteristics of the groups. Sanua's study gives ample evidence of this fact. He discovered many other relationships besides those we have mentioned. One of these is particularly interesting, as it confirms Durkheim's findings: 40 per cent of the Protestant paranoid patients had suicidal tendencies, compared with 20 per cent of the Jewish paranoid patients; the Catholics on the contrary tended to be more outwardly aggressive and impulsive, depending on the ethnic group (homicidal tendencies were stronger among the Irish than among the Italians).

The conclusions that can be drawn from this analysis are that the values and norms that make up the religious culture of an ethnic group are of prime importance in the aetiology of mental illness: the family factor is determined by ethno-religious cultural traditions. However, there are variations in these values and norms according to social class, although there would appear to be fewer variations in the Jewish than in the Protestant group. On this last point we can say nothing about the Catholic group, since all the Catholic schizophrenics in Sanua's study belonged to the lower class.

Religious experience, or the application of religious principles to everyday life, has nothing to do with this type of study. Sanua states emphatically that signs of psychic conflict caused by religious identification were very infrequent among the population he studied; in the rare cases where it occurred, the interest in religion came after the illness rather than before and was only temporary. We need therefore to turn to different sources of information to measure the impact of religious experience and to find out whether Durkheim's hypothesis that it has an integrative value can be confirmed.

2 Mental disorder and religious experience

Is the religious service a communion of the faithful participating in a mystical experience, or is it merely, like the Catholic *tenebrae*, a ritual full of pathos marking the descent into the night? Can religion help man to transcend his psychic conflicts by giving life a meaning, as was the opinion of Jung, who called religion the royal road to mental health? Or is it merely an outgrowth on the organism of life, a morbid proliferation of cells? Let us see whether we can discover the answers to these questions.

Religious experience seems to be a topic of more vital concern today to the psychiatrist and the priest than the question of mere religious affiliation, which we dealt with earlier. From the Jewish point of view, Baruk has often emphasized the importance in the causation of mental disorder of the gap between our present-day social behaviour and the laws of the Ten Commandments, which creates increasing insecurity in the individual. From the Catholic point of view, the founding of Choisy's journal, *Psyché*, was an attempt to provide a meeting-point for the priest and the psychiatrist. Their co-operation is necessary, for example, when the priest discovers that the scruples of a confessant are more than a wish to be morally pure, to come nearer to God, and may be a sign of pathological tendencies that need the help of a psychiatrist. Similarly, the psychiatrist can often achieve a cure by asking the priest to work side by side with him in rehabilitating the patient. In Italy there has been some concern to verify the genuineness of the vocations of future priests, and there have been long discussions on whether or not to use psychological tests. On the Protestant side, Bergman emphasizes the part religion can play in psycho-therapy,[16] Tiébout has no doubt about its importance in treating cases of alcoholism,[17] while Frankl considers the repression or decline of our spiritual life to be the real pathology of our time.[18]

Every religion has its ethos. Should we emphasize the communal aspect of religion, as Durkheim did for suicide and Dayton for mental illness? Should we think in terms of a continuum between collectivity-oriented and individualistic religions? Or ought we to take the analysis further and examine dogma, ritual and ethics? The statement has often been made, but with no facts to substantiate it, that the absence of confession in the Protestant religion produces an obsession with sin and an acute feeling of guilt, resulting in inhibitory states. In sects where confession is accepted, but where it is public and not secret, it is said to encourage exhibitionism. On the other hand, many psychiatrists have found more disturb-ances among Catholics than among Protestants, precisely because of confession: the Catholic who has not admitted everything to the priest and has received absolution on top of a lie will be more likely to end up in mental hospital than the Protestant who is tormented by not being able to confess. It is possible that the Jewish belief in a pact between the people of Israel and their God is more relevant to mental health than the intense community spirit of the Jews. Of course, the community feelings are there, and divine protection embraces the whole people (except in cases of collective and not individual lack of belief). But it is possible that the hope or the conviction of this support from God, by transcending it, strengthens the solidarity which is the only thing the sociologists considered.

We cannot really discuss these points and other related ones here:

they are pure interpretations, based, no doubt, on clinical impressions, but not substantiated by reliable enough data.

There are three types of data available on the role of religion:

(1) The small sample of patients has been used by some psychiatrists. For example: out of 68 cases of psychosis in a hospital in rural Kentucky, more than half (51·5 per cent) showed no signs of having been influenced by religion; 20·5 per cent of the psychoses were coloured by religion, but without it being clear whether or not religion was a causative factor; 17·2 per cent were an expression of the individual's revolt against his childhood faith, but a more detailed analysis showed that this revolt was merely a rationalization of the parent-child conflict. Finally, in 10·3 per cent of the cases the patient had tried to find an answer to his problems in religion, and his failure to do so was the cause of his breakdown.[19]

Oates found among future Baptist missionaries in the South of the U.S.A. many cases of emotional frustration and of conflict with parents. However, the students were shielded from psychosis by their religious way of life, the good priest replacing the cruel father and the Church community creating a climate of security which gradually dispelled their anxiety. On the basis of 76 clinical observations in Louisville, the same author suggested that religion has a twofold effect, both negative (the obsession with sin, the importance of taboos against drinking, dancing and sexual relations creating a state of anxiety in some patients) and positive: religion, and especially prayer, has a soothing effect, reassures the mind, comforts the patient and relieves anxiety.

From these various studies it is possible to conclude that religion in itself is less important than the individual's response to it— whether he accepts it, rebels against it or fails in his quest for the divine. In the second place, religion counts less than the way in which it has been taught by the father or mother. The bias introduced by the parents means that it is parent-child relations that affect the mental health of the individual, in the guise of religious practices and beliefs. Finally, the religious way of life is more important as a therapeutic aid than as an explanatory factor in mental disorder.[20]

(2) The study of religious sects constitutes the second main area of research. We mentioned Eaton and Weil's study of the Hutterite colonies in Canada and the U.S.A., which aimed at evaluating the effect of life in an isolated community on mental health. These are religious communities; their cohesion comes essentially from their mystical values. We saw that in spite of appearances to the contrary, psychosis and neurosis are not unknown in these communities, but they are less severe and more often latent than overt. We need now to examine the part played by religion among the

Hutterites. Religion goes a long way towards explaining the paradoxical character of their morbidity when compared with the U.S.A. in general: the almost total absence of organic psychosis, since alcohol, drugs and sexual indulgence are forbidden; the very small number of schizophrenics, the high rate of manic depressives and the rarity of severe forms of neurosis. Eaton and Weil show that the pious atmosphere, the prayers and the brotherly love permeating the settlements eliminate doubt and anxiety and create a feeling of security. The conclusion is the same as the one we reached earlier: the effect is therapeutic rather than aetiological. We could now add that it is preventive. However, any disturbance that occurs is structured by the religious values, which explains why the Hutterites, in contrast to the secularized North Americans, are more prone to depression than anxiety: this is only a pathological reflection of the cyclical rhythm of religious life, with its periods of spiritual aridity followed by periods of mystical exaltation.[21] Oates comes to similar conclusions: sects are closed communities protecting their members against mental disorder; out of 173 patients studied by Southard, only 4 per cent were members of religious sects. Although it may seem, on the contrary, that sects have a morbid character, this is because in most cases the focal point of their faith is inspiration from the Holy Ghost; this inspirational character (deliberate inducement of trances, baptism by the Holy Ghost, glossolalia, etc.) gives what are merely cultural phenomena the appearance of 'clinical' ones. We put forward a similar argument ourselves against medical men on the subject of ecstatic states of possession in Afro-Brazilian religions. However, it seems necessary to differentiate between sects: some have a positive protective function; others have a negative effect in that they intensify the psychic conflict between the desire for absolute perfection and the instincts—particularly the sexual instinct. In some cases they foster rigid attitudes by their reaction against all involvement in 'worldly' activities. Finally, they tend to take under their wing (especially in the case of the esoteric urban sects which are multiplying today in our big cities) all sorts of anxious and depressed people, individuals who have been broken by industrial society. They can be veritable breeding-grounds for psychiatric disorder, which they tend to exalt, whereas the conventional Churches control and repress manifestations of disturbance. Psychiatrists in Brazil have shown the part played by spiritualism in the development of mental disorder (although they have tended to exaggerate the problem somewhat). In France, Chombart de Lauwe, Colinon, Delay and others have also drawn attention to this last characteristic of sects.[22]

(3) Finally, we have a series of case studies illustrating various religious ways of life, some of which are conducive to mental

disturbance and others far removed from it. Certain styles of religious life are regressive and pathological, while others are progressive and produce healthy personalities.

Oates[23] arrived at this conclusion through studying the religious interpretations contained in his patients' delusions. He found evidence of an obsession with sin, a rigid condemnation of sexual aberrations (such as the self-condemnation of the patient who in intercourse with his wife saw her as a prostitute), a fear of others in patients who crystallize a 'legalistic' structure around the real or imaginary hostility of other people, a confusion of the self with God (for example, in patients who imagine they are crucified like Christ), and Messianic day-dreams in patients who seek an escape from anxiety by cutting themselves off from the disturbing outer world. He was also able to differentiate a religion of hostility (rebellious sects), a religion of dependence (this was the religion Freud was thinking of when he described God as a father-figure), a religion of spiritual aridity and, finally, a religion of the spirit, the only valid form of religion. McKenzie[24] has mainly analysed three of these types: 'legalistic' religion, which is essentially prohibitive and takes the form of a neurotic perfectionism related to the stern Biblical superego; a religion of dependence which is basically the reverse side of a latent rebelliousness that is being resisted in the name of Christian ethics; it corresponds to a neurotic conflict and fear of freedom, with negativistic and compulsive tendencies (the religious equivalent of the type of personality found in totalitarian political parties); finally, a religion of the spirit: religious belief, far from being conducive to repression and dissociation, on the contrary integrates the inclinations, feelings and ideas of the individual and focuses his activity on love for others. It should by now be obvious that illness or health come first and religion afterwards. Religion can be transformed by neurotics into a pathological construction; it can nourish the delusions of psychotics, but religion does not create either form of mental disorder.

Now that we have reached the end of this chapter it is easier to see what prompted the dialogue between psychiatrists and clergymen of different religions. On the one hand they must preserve religion from parasitic elements produced by family conflicts or the inhumanity of industrial society, which can infiltrate into religion and turn it into a neurotic phenomenon. On the other hand, they must foster the particular aspects of the Church, such as community spirit and discipline, which provide a regulating influence on emotional life, a spiritual education and a guidance towards a saner existence.

VII   The psychiatry of social groups: II. Ethnic groups

American studies of religious groups do not make any distinction between ethnic and religious group, so that it is difficult to separate the effect of the two factors. Even if religion is not practised nor even recognized, it shapes popular culture from generation to generation, and its implicit rules underlie the customs of a people, especially where child-rearing is concerned. Faith may well die, but culture becomes its death-mask. Therefore in this chapter we shall deal with ethnic groups, not as cultural groups, but as minority groups. We live in a particularly mobile world, where whole sections of the population move from country to country and even from one continent to another. Claudel once described America as the new kind of Paschal table where different races, Indians, Negroes descended from slaves, whites from the most diverse countries, Spaniards, Portuguese, Italians, Poles, Lebanese, etc., commune in sharing the same work and the same bread. But other countries besides America are melting-pots. To mention only one European country, France seems to be rapidly becoming a nation of executives directing an army of foreigners from Poles to North Africans, who do the menial work. We ought to ask ourselves what effect this mixing of peoples can have on mental health.[1]

Figures compiled by Laughlin a long time ago and quoted by Klineberg show the differential incidence of mental disorder among various ethnic groups in the U.S.A.: native-born whites, native-born whites of foreign parentage and immigrants.[2] The figures show the ratio of insanity to the proportion which each group constitutes of the total population of the U.S.A.

Apart from a few cases, such as the Japanese and the Swiss, the proportion of mentally-ill foreigners is consistently higher than that of non-migrants. Stonequist pointed out that immigrants in the

139

Table 18 Incidence of insanity among immigrant groups (% of quota fulfilled)

Native-born whites (both parents native to U.S.A.) . . 73

„   „   „   (one foreign parent) 104

„   „   „   (two foreign parents) 108

Japanese	42	Dutch	171
Swiss	69	Greeks	172
Chinese	78	Germans	174
Rumanians	100	Portuguese	181
Canadians	124	Scandinavians	193
Austro-Hungarians	134	Turks	200
Mexicans	137	Russians, Finns, Poles . .	265
English	156	Bulgarians	300
Italians	157	Irish	305
French	158	Serbs	400

U.S.A. show a rate of hospitalization for mental disorder two to three times as high as the rate in their native country.[3] Thus it is not some racial characteristic which is responsible for these high figures, but the move from one country to another. Laughlin's mental-disorder rate for foreigners was 225·26 per 100,000 population, compared with 73·27 for native Americans; in the countries of origin of these foreigners the rate at the same period was only 193·36 for north-western Europe and 188·50 for eastern Europe.[4]

However, these figures can be criticized.[5] The rate for white Americans is drawn from the whole of the U.S.A., including rural areas, small provincial towns and large cities; we have seen that, according to hospitalization figures, there are fewer cases of mental disorder in the country and in small towns than in large cities. Now, immigrants are mainly concentrated in the big industrial cities, where there are many more treatment facilities; often they are unmarried, and when they become ill have no other recourse than hospitalization. These facts probably partly explain the high hospitalization rate among immigrants. Other factors are sex and age. There are more mentally-ill men and women in the U.S.A., especially in the 15–25-year-old age-group; not only are most immigrants men, but as they are usually young people starting a new life, they are mainly in this age-group. Laughlin took these criticisms into account and later standardized his figures on the basis of the population aged 20 and over, which reduced the rate among foreigners to 34·9. Yet other corrections are needed. The figures we quoted are based on the total number of hospitalized patients. The length of hospitalization varies according to the psychosis. Therefore at any given date we are faced with a back-log of chronic schizophrenic or paranoid patients who have remained in hospital without treatment for long periods. It is therefore necessary to look at first admissions only, when the picture changes yet again. For example, in New York State, over a period of three years (1929–31), out of 26,765 first admissions, we find 15,704 native-born Americans (58·7 per 100,000 population) and 10,987 foreigners (here the rate is only 115·1 per 100,000). If we correct for differences due to sex and age, the gap is narrowed still further: the rates become 91·8 for native-born Americans and 108·8 for foreigners. Moreover, hospitalized patients are mainly from the underprivileged sector of society; Americans from the upper-middle and upper classes tend to be treated in private nursing-homes or at home. Since immigrants tend to belong to the lower social strata, we have good reason to think that, if class factors were controlled, the differences would cease to be significant. Malzberg maintains that if the uncorrected figures are considered, there is an excess of foreigners over natives of 96 per cent; if the figures are corrected for sex and age, the excess is reduced to 19 per cent, and if the ecological factor is taken into account—that is, if one eliminates wealthy areas where there are no foreigners—the gap is reduced to 8 per cent. Do more recent studies confirm these findings?

In 1932 Ødegaard studied Norwegian immigrants in Minnesota, and found that during the previous forty years the Norwegians had had a higher rate of hospitalization than Americans born in Minnesota and Norwegians in Norway. But when in 1945 he studied the same problem again (the effects of geographic mobility in Norway), he found, contrary to all expectations, that immigrants had a lower rate of hospitalization than non-migrants. It seems as if there are two types of mobility, 'internal' (as mentioned in our chapter on ecology) and 'external' (from country to country), both having different effects.[6] In collaboration with Lee, Malzberg made a second study of hospitalized patients in New York for the period 1939–41. He concluded that the length of time the immigrants had been in the U.S.A. was the most important factor: the greater number of hospitalized foreigners was due to the fact that first admissions are much more frequent among recent immigrants than among earlier immigrants and the native population combined.[7] That is to say, once the upheaval of being transplanted is over and the initial trauma is overcome the immigrants' morbidity rate falls within the average range for the population as a whole. There still remains a last element to consider in explaining the higher rates among immigrants. Could it be that people who emigrate are already disturbed or predisposed to disturbance? Is migration only the search for a better life, a wanderlust that could be the sign of incipient mental disorder? This point is emphasized by many South American psychiatrists, who recommend a stricter check on the mental health of immigrants entering their countries. It is, of course, very difficult to control this variable. It is easier to evaluate its importance in relation to internal migration: Keeler and Vitols estimated that 14 per cent of the Negro schizophrenic population of North Carolina show these particular traits.[8]

It would thus appear that, since research techniques have become more refined, the gap between U.S.A. nationals and members of ethnic minorities is still evident, but is much smaller than it seemed at first.

Studies made in France, where this field has been of particular interest to sociologists and psychiatrists,[9] confirm the American findings. First of all, foreigners show a higher rate of hospitalized mental illness than the French population, and their rate of mental disorder is higher than that of their corresponding native countries. This is true even where the immigrants have settled very near their country of origin, as with the Italians in Nice. However, regional differences and ecological factors must be taken into account. The highest concentrations of hospitalized immigrants are found in the urban centres; where immigrants have settled on the land, as in the Gers region, there is virtually no difference in the figures between native and migrant populations, as though close ties to the earth counteracted the ill-effects of being uprooted. A second factor that must be considered is whether the immigrants are dispersed or concentrated in communities that faithfully keep up their cultural traditions. In the second case the stable, organized group is well protected against the pathogenic effects of transplantation, as if the migrants had created an extension of their country of origin. They are still really living at home, as we saw earlier in the case of the Dutch settlements in France.[10] The traumatic impact of arrival in a new country and the consequent necessity of distinguishing between the newly arrived and the older immigrants is well illustrated by Daumezon and his collaborators in the case of North Africans. The North African usually experiences a crisis within six months of his arrival in France; once this critical period is over, he tends to adjust to his new surroundings.[11] On the other hand, Pélicier observed among the French settlers who fled to France after Algerian independence a 'primary crisis' with traumatic reactions (stupor, anxiety, depression, inconsistent behaviour) quite different from the secondary psychological reactions occurring later and only in a small number of subjects.[12] Finally, French psychiatrists, while recognizing the effects of a sudden change of surroundings, have drawn attention to the predisposition of the subjects before they leave their own country. Many uprooted people are already poorly adjusted to their original environment, and a change of country can be an attempt at resolving their conflicts.[13] It is very hard, both in France and the U.S.A., to make an effective study of this particular variable. However, when examining the files of immigrant patients from Guadeloupe and Martinique, the author has very often come across references to hospitalization or untreated disorders prior to arrival in France. In France, as in the United States, there are naturally variations from one ethnic group to another. The greater the cultural gap between the original background and the new environment, the greater the chance of mental disorder. The importance of this gap can even be seen in internal migration (cf. Le Guillant and Torrubia's study of Breton maids working in Paris, which showed a differential rate of disturbance according to whether the girls came from the Armor or the Arcoat region). There is even more reason for there to be a difference between foreigners: the rate of hospitalization is three times as great among West Africans in France as among European immigrants.[14]

There appears to be a special psychiatry of transplanted and uprooted people. What are its particular characteristics? Statistics quoted by Malzberg give the rates per 100,000 population for New York State as shown in Table 19.

Some of these differences are due to the differential age composition of the two groups: if age is controlled, there are no significant differences for alcoholic psychosis and general paresis. Other discrepancies are due to cultural factors: immigrants do not totally and immediately change their old habits, they retain them in their new home and cling to them as though to their lost country. Alcoholism can, of course, be a panic reaction to change; but we must note that it is usually found only among certain groups and is therefore a cultural trait. Among the Irish 18 per cent of all psychosis is due to alcohol, among Scandinavians 6·6 per cent, and in the U.S.A. as a whole only 3 per cent. The proof that it is really a cultural feature is that, as assimilation of American values occurs, the rate begins to fall: among second-generation Irish the percentage of psychosis caused in this way is 9·4 and in Scandinavians 2·8, whereas Italians, who are ordinarily continent people, pick up the habit of drinking in their new country, with the result that the second generation shows an increase in alcoholic psychosis from 0·2 per cent of all psychosis to 1·2 per cent.

Table 19 Mental disorder and ethnic origin, New York State

	Native-born	Foreign-born
Senile psychosis	4·8	12·1
Cerebral arteriosclerosis	7·3	18·2
General paresis	5·1	12·1
Alcoholic psychosis	3·2	7·4
Manic-depressive psychosis	8·2	14·9
Schizophrenia	15·2	30·2

Clearly, it is not enough to contrast non-migrants with migrants. We must examine each ethnic group separately in order to discover its particular pattern of morbidity. According to Malzberg's figures, the Irish show the highest rates of first admissions for senile psychosis and alcoholic psychosis, and the lowest for general paresis. The Scandinavians have the second highest rate of morbidity, also with a high proportion of alcoholic psychosis and in addition a high rate of general paresis. Germans, Italians and English come next. The same psychosis can take on different forms according to the ethnic group. Opler's research on schizophrenia in Irish and Italian immigrants and in Americans shows that in the Italian group personal prestige is an important factor.[15] Sanua notes differences in pathology due to popular attitudes to sex. The Irish link sex with sin, while the Italians have a much more permissive attitude: this is reflected in guilt-feelings in the Irish that are not found among the Italians.[16] Opler and Singer contrast the passive character of schizophrenia in the Irish with the aggressive and impulsive nature of the illness among Italians, a reflection on the pathological level of the introverted nature of the former and the outgoing temperament of the latter.[17] In our own work at the São Paulo Mental Hospital in Brazil, we came across a surprising predominance of catatonic schizophrenia among the Japanese, in contrast to the paranoid forms found among Spaniards. We believe this is due to the opposite character of the two cultures, the Japanese tendency to repress outward signs of emotion and what one might call the quixotic temperament of the Spaniards.

In France Koechlin introduced a time dimension instead of the ethnic dimension. Immigrants show successive stages of disturbance irrespective of their national origin. He found highly atypical depressive states in subjects who had only been in the country a short while (from a few months to two or three years at most), accompanied by irritability and a tendency to take refuge in alcoholism. A second stage can then evolve from this depressed state in the form of hysterical neurosis or hypochondriacal delusions: 'The anxiety created by the feeling of being different from other people finds a solution in the possibility of withdrawal from society which illness represents.' The commonest third stage takes the form of systematized delusions of interpretation and persecution, when the patient does not in fact feel persecuted by the whole of French society, nor by the government or police (except for some old Russian refugees who see communists everywhere), but usually by colleagues and neighbours, or, if he is married, by his wife's family.[18] Stanciu, who also studied migrants in general, without reference to their origin, distinguishes three or four different disorders typical of migrants: certain forms of pseudo-deficiency, paranoid and vindictive attitudes, anxiety, and depression which sometimes goes as far as suicide.[19] Boitelle, who studied an extremely heterogeneous hospital population, found no significant differences between the disturbances found among Italians, Poles, Moroccans, Hungarians and Yugoslavs; nearly all the patients showed the same psychotic confusion, breaking out shortly after their arrival in France, and disappearing rapidly if they are not hospitalized.[20, 21]

It is interesting to speculate why the Americans are more concerned with ethnic differences than the French. Obviously the scientific climate in the two countries is very different. America being the home of cultural anthropology, more attention will be paid there to the effect of different national cultures. France, on the other hand, is the home of sociology, and therefore the emphasis will be placed on the general phenomenon of migration. Another factor to be considered is that psychoanalysis has been much more readily accepted and has had a much deeper effect in the U.S.A.

than in France; this has led the Americans—as we shall see later —to search for the fundamental causes of psychosis in the methods of child-rearing in the immigrants' native countries—in other words, to study individual subjects. In France there is more interest in the social situation to which the foreigner has to adjust; explanations are sought more in external influences than in the cultural background of the immigrant. This brings us to the problem of interpreting the data we have just briefly summarized.

Let us start with the more psychoanalytically-oriented interpretations and move towards the more sociological ones.

Some psychoanalysts regard moving as a situation which reactivates the original anxiety of the child's first move away from the mother, when he leaves her side and takes his first steps. Separation from the mother is not experienced as freedom, but as a feeling of being deserted by the protective figure. The anxiety reawakened by migration is much more traumatic than the original anxiety, because the desertion by the mother country is made legal: all the formalities the immigrant has to go through to be able to live and work in a new country mark the severing of the 'umbilical cord', the new process of 'weaning', of leaving the mother's side. What is more, the new country appears as a 'wicked stepmother', the 'bad mother' who has replaced the good one. The man who has left home with no hope of returning desires to be adopted by this new mother, but he also has doubts that generate a feeling of inner panic: Will she accept him? In addition to this, the immigrant can regress, as a result of the cultural shock, to the Oedipal stage: the policeman or the boss takes on the role of a restrictive father or even of a sadistic, castrating one. Any effort to integrate him into the value-system of the new country will be experienced as phallic or anal aggression. This is particularly disturbing for those who have not been able to reconstruct a community life that keeps the traditional values of the native land (representing the intimate bliss and security of the mother's breast). This sort of interpretation offers food for thought, but we will not dwell on it here. It contains elements that are undoubtedly valid: one does not usually sleep well in a strange bed, or in a hotel room while travelling, owing to the awakening in the unconscious of the primitive anxiety of being separated from the mother. But we must limit our field to sociological issues.

Our second approach is also psychoanalytic, but it relates more to sociology: it studies the differences in child-rearing, socialization and parental discipline according to ethnic origin. There are several good American studies in this field—for example, the work of Barrabee and Von Mering.[22] They show that in Irish families the tie with the mother is very strong, especially in girls, but this affection is accompanied by strict discipline which is supervised by the father. This produces a puritanical attitude and a general acceptance of repressions, with the result that the Irish, as we mentioned earlier, grow up with feelings of guilt and are tormented by the idea of sexual sin. The Italians in the U.S.A., especially the southern Italians, have retained the typical Mediterranean patriarchal family: the father punishes, controls, manages; the mother reacts against the father's severity by being doubly affectionate to the child—in other words, by becoming an over-protective mother. According to Barrabee and Von Mering, this could be the clue to the origin of schizophrenia among Italians. In fact, it was noted by Frazee that schizophrenia occurs mainly in families where fathers are severely cruel and rejecting.[23] Sperling found that in a group of Italian patients 60 per cent showed hostile attitudes to their fathers and 50 per cent to their mothers; in a group of Irish patients he found hostile attitudes towards the father and ambivalent ones towards the mother.[24] Sanua compared the families of schizophrenic patients: he discovered more over-protection by Italian parents and more rejection by Irish parents; however, other characteristics found among Italian fathers were violence, lack of self-control and domineering and brutal behaviour, while the main problem in the Irish fathers was chronic alcoholism. The Irish mothers were often domestic workers or were in poorly paid jobs, while most of the Italian mothers stayed at home. These facts play an important part in creating mental disorder and in determining its subsequent course; they affect its aetiology as well as its semiology.[25]

However, these parent-child relations which have such serious effects on the psyche are determined by the culture of the group. It is therefore possible to consider them, from a different viewpoint, as processes of socialization—that is, transmission of values and formation of the basic personality. Research done in the U.S.A. has been concerned with children brought up outside the country of their parents' origin; what we are interested in for the moment is what happens to immigrants brought up in their own country and suddenly experiencing transplantation into a new world. Surely the fundamental event here is the cultural shock? The family background of the immigrant is only significant in so far as it explains the differences in basic personality structure. This brings us to a third interpretation, in terms of the acculturation process.[26] We are reminded of the famous French debate on migration between André Gide and Maurice Barrès known as the 'poplar controversy' because it uses the analogy of the cutting that produces a new tree. Barrès emphasized the negative effect of uprooting people, while

Gide regarded this process as an essential condition of creative originality. Both are right, of course, but it depends on the individual. Strong personalities grow richer in the process; acculturation alone can account for the progress of man; however, it always involves a crisis which for some is difficult to surmount.

The learning of new cultural patterns, as Koechlin points out, is never easy once the malleable childhood stage is over. The attempt to adjust is a strain for the adult and often results in failure. The new environment that he cannot master is experienced as hostile, even if it is not really so. This is why Duchêne, for example, regards social and economic influence as insignificant. Among the indigenous French there are people of exactly the same socioeconomic level as the migrant who are free from these particular disturbances. Thus the essential factor is not the strange environment in itself, but the experience of strangeness. In the same way, Le Guillant considers that it is not the economic and social conditions (physical environment, work, etc.) that upset the transplanted person, at least not directly. Their influence is mediated either by affective phenomena (homesickness characterized by depression and withdrawal into passive resignation) or, more important, by the experience of a 'contradiction' (the migrant perceives his new surroundings not as different but as a contradiction of his original environment; he is both attracted and repelled by them) and by 'alienation' (the migrant perceives himself as 'alienated', separate from other people, isolated, excluded from the group into which he is supposed to integrate; he cannot establish the sort of communication with others which alone can disalienate and fulfil the individual).[27] Finally, Sivadon maintains that migration is pathogenic only if it creates a substantial gap between the original culture and the new institutions, and if the subject's basic personality pattern remains unchanged.[28]

French authors have obviously tended to emphasize the importance of the gap between basic personality and new cultural environment. The Americans have not neglected this aspect (cf. Ruesch, who shows that acculturation is marked by frustration: the responses the subject has inherited from his original culture are inappropriate, and this results in anxiety and hostility). But they have been more interested to show the changes occurring in the personality as new values and norms are assimilated. Stonequist's *The Marginal Man* is entirely devoted to this aspect of the problem. During a first period, straight after migration, the individual is removed from the control of his original society; he is freed from the old restrictions, but has not yet begun to experience the new ones. This can bring about a release of asocial and amoral tendencies. As the migrant adjusts to his new environment, he is reshaped

by it; but this does not mean that the effects of his original formation are destroyed. His self is split in half; there are two different
people warring in his innermost being. This is the crucial period
that holds the key to the origin of mental disorder in migrants: the
conflict between two cultures is experienced, not as an outside
phenomenon (a conflict between the basic personality and the new
environment), but as an inner struggle between two identities in
mutual contradiction. The conflict takes place within the individual
between his old and his new personality: hence the disturbance in
his mental equilibrium.

We do not think the two approaches are contradictory but
rather that they complement each other. The important point is to
distinguish between primary and secondary crises. In the former,
the conflict between basic personality and new environment
effectively takes place outside the person, with the added complica-
tion of linguistic isolation[29] and the syndrome of homesickness:

> which comes from the loss of habitual horizons and the absence
> of familiar people and things. At home, beings and objects,
> buildings and landscapes, are reference-points that reassure
> us and give us our bearings. . . . But I cannot see the new
> surroundings in relation to myself, because there are no familiar
> landmarks to help me apprehend and digest the whole.
> Minkowski and his disciple Solanes have made a remarkable
> analysis of the devaluation and distortion of time in the
> experience of exile.[30]

In the later, secondary phase of disturbance, the dominant feature
is no longer the conflict between the individual and the environment, but the marginality of the individual: he is both the same and
a different person; part of his being belongs to the old world and
part to the new. The syndromes found in this secondary stage are
instability caused by loyalty to two conflicting groups, ambivalent
attitudes, a feeling of hopelessness at being pulled in opposite
directions, the inability to create a synthesis, an increase in
emotionality, hypersensitivity, etc. Some individuals will naturally
resort to compensatory mechanisms, but in such a climate of
anxiety these mechanisms will still be morbid, and will tend to
take the form of a disguising of feelings, withdrawal and flight into
personal fantasy.

The culturally oriented approach is not incompatible with the
psychoanalytic approach we discussed earlier; some authors have
combined the two successfully. An example is the study made by
Prange of a Chinese immigrant girl, where he shows the effect of
the clash between basic personality and new environment. The girl's
personality structure was adequate in her own country, but not in

149

the U.S.A., where she was separated from her family and her habitual work-situation, and where her idea of love was not accepted. She experienced these frustrations as a lack of oral gratification. In fact, Prange emphasizes the general oral character of the frustrations of immigrants: home represents early childhood, the warmth of the mother's breast, the pleasures of feeling and sucking; separation from the 'mother' country rekindles the desire for gratification; it is therefore not surprising to find that foreigners often react to homesickness by boulimia or anorexia, and alcoholism tends to be the most frequent form of disorder.[31] Thus, to be really meaningful, the study of mental disorder in migrants should be seen in terms of Mauss's concept of the 'total social phenomenon' and of the interpretation of this concept by Gurvitch in his 'depth sociology'. In other words, there are superimposed strata which the psychiatrist must examine one by one to arrive at a comprehensive interpretation.

But precisely because psychoses—and neuroses caused by problems of adjustment—are total phenomena, we must take into account both their cultural and their social dimensions. Minority groups can also be oppressed groups. The Negro in the United States is an example that led Kardiner to produce his superb analysis of the 'mark of oppression'. Many traits found in the oppressed Negro (escape into alcoholism or vice, lowering of intelligence under the stultifying influence of a hostile environment, frequent self-destructive responses on the Rorschach test) can naturally be found in other communities suffering from segregation.[32] But even where segregation is minimal, the migrant is still in a competitive world where he feels alone and unsupported in his struggle. Sexual competition often reduces him to the company of prostitutes and women of low reputation, competition in the labour market leaves him with the jobs the natives refuse because they consider them inferior; he is thus the first to become unemployed when there is an economic crisis. Finally, ecological competition pushes him into areas of social disintegration in large cities, or squatter settlements in the suburbs.[33] The influence of social factors is brought clearly into focus in Boitelle's study of immigrant patients in a hospital in the Moselle Département. These immigrants could not speak French; they were isolated, undernourished (they sent the best part of their wages back to their family) and badly housed; they lived in a region where twenty-seven nationalities rubbed shoulders; they were constantly subjected to bureaucratic formalities, despised by their French workmates, ill-adapted to industrial work, most of them having been agricultural workers. Often, as in the case of the Poles, they received no news from home.[34] In other words, even if a person emigrates to improve his social status, he will first of all experience a drop in status—and we have seen the role of downward social mobility in the aetiology of mental illness. The same pathogenic factors we discussed in the previous chapters are present here: the unfavourable ecological situation and the lower social status; but when a person has been uprooted from his own country their negative effect is infinitely increased.

In the case of second-generation immigrants it seems that the situation should be less traumatic. However, Thomas and Znaniecki's study, *The Polish Peasant in Europe and America*, showed that conflicts can be even more serious for the children than for the parents. When the child goes to school he becomes to a great extent acculturated, but in addition to the influence of the school he is influenced by his parents, who tend to react to transplantation by idealizing their lost country; their efforts are directed, especially in the case of the mother, who is more traditionally oriented than the father, towards maintaining in their offspring the values of the native country. The child finds himself torn between two conflicting cultures: that of the family (or the street, if he lives in an immigrant neighbourhood) and that of the school. Two things can happen: either the child acts as a mediator between his non-acculturated family and the new environment, when he becomes conscious of his important role, evades parental control and becomes a rebel. (Criminals are found in this first group.) Or else he is pampered and over-protected, in which case he becomes permanently maladjusted. Research by American psychoanalysts shows that too close a tie with the mother can hinder the Americanization of foreign-born males.[35] In the case of mixed marriages, where the parents come from different cultural backgrounds, each parent strives to draw the child into his or her own culture. There follows the interiorization of a dual system of conflicting norms, which intensifies the child's marginality. The author studied a sample of problem children in São Paulo and found a higher percentage of disturbance in bilingual families, even where the only language spoken in the family was the foreign language. McBee found that, out of 102 students with personality disorders, 57 per cent had a foreign mother and 47 per cent had a foreign father, compared with 30 per cent whose parents were both foreign. It is, of course, possible to argue that mixed marriages are particularly unstable and often end in separation, so that we could be dealing with another factor here, the 'broken home'. But this is not the case: in McBee's sample we find only 40 per cent broken homes compared with percentages for unbroken homes of 57·47 per cent (for one foreign parent out of two) and 30 per cent (both parents foreign). The cause of disturbance would therefore not reside in conflict within the family itself, but in the conflict between cultures.[36] Terashima also showed, in his study of three schizophrenic second-generation Japanese immigrants in Canada, the importance of intergenerational conflict in causing mental disturbance in the off-spring.[37]

However, these studies can be criticized on one ground: they do not use control groups. It is therefore not surprising that other studies have produced different results. Malzberg investigated mental disorder in American children of foreign parentage: he found that, barring two exceptions (younger families and families of more recent immigration), these children showed higher percentages of disorder than American-born adults and their children, but lower percentages than foreign adults. He concludes that, since the 'racial' element is probably constant from one generation to another, this proves that the environmental factor plays the most important part in the genesis of mental disorder. The child of foreign parentage who is born in the U.S.A. is already better adapted to the American way of life, and therefore less vulnerable, than his parents.[38]

In our opinion, as people become more and more acculturated so the chances of morbidity decrease. Hinkle and Wolff's study covered three generations: it appeared that at least by the third generation the families had climbed from the slums to the respectable or middle-class residential districts, from elementary schooling to higher education, and from unskilled to skilled work. At this point it is possible to state that integration into the new society is complete. The ethnic factor no longer intervenes as a social factor.[39]

VIII   The psychiatry of social groups: III. The family

The reader may have noticed that so far our discussions have always led back to the family. It is the opinion of many psychiatrists that, whatever the factor considered, whether it be ecological area, social class, religion or ethnic group, it always operates through the medium of the family and childhood experience. We shall therefore end this study of social influence with the family group.

The family can be studied from two different points of view. First of all, it may be regarded as a structured social institution, controlled by the State through the registration of marriage, or by the Church, which regards the marital bond as indissoluble. Even where the State accepts divorce, the marriage contract is not broken freely: the separation must be accompanied by guarantees and given an official seal. This is the way Durkheim and most French sociologists view the family. It can also be seen as a social group that structures, according to particular cultural norms, a set of relations between husband and wife, parents and children, brothers and sisters, and eventually grandparents, parents and grandchildren. This is the predominant point of view of American sociologists. Thus there are two ways in which the family can be studied, either as an institution or as a set of personal relations.

1   The psychiatry of the family from the institutional viewpoint

The first statistical studies of mental disorder which always took marital status into account clearly revealed that some status groups were more particularly vulnerable to personality disorders than others. Rates for the U.S.A. in 1923 are shown in Table 20.

The greater frequency of psychotic disorders among the un-married is often explained in terms of the sexual frustration of adolescents. Marriage brings sexual security to the couple.[1] We feel

Table 20 Rate of mental disorder according to marital status

	Per 100,000 population	
	Men	*Women*
Married	170·9	255·9
Unmarried	292·7	189·3
Widowed	428·2	423·0
Divorced	1,112·5	1,120·3

that Durkheim's point of view is more reasonable: these statistical findings, which are so similar to the findings on suicide, come within the scope of the sociology of mental pathology, which we outlined earlier with reference to *The Division of Labour in Society*. Marriage not only regulates sexual life, but creates intimate relationships of social co-operation. In so doing, it controls the individual's emotional life and helps him towards an equilibrium lacking in the unmarried state. If single women are less prone to disturbance than married women, as these figures show, this is because they have much closer family ties and are much more integrated into their parental family than young men. Marriage creates serious difficulties for them: they have to learn to take the initiative, play new roles, manage the home, etc. These unfamiliar problems can have traumatic effects. On the other hand, the family constitutes a protective environment, and the severing of the marital tie, whether by death or divorce, is more detrimental to mental health than the fact of being unmarried. This is as true for suicide as it is for psychosis.

More recent figures given by Malzberg for hospitalized patients in New York State confirm the previous ones. The pattern of first admissions from 1929 to 1931 for the population aged fifteen and over is given in Table 21.

However, there is no longer any difference between the number of males and females in each marital status group. As Katherine Bement Davis pointed out, marriage is as valid an aid to mental health for women as it is for men.[2] Malzberg found two exceptions to this: syphilitic psychosis and alcoholic psychosis. Single women show less paresis than men because women tend to be infected by their husbands; and, in spite of the relaxation in moral stan-

154

dards, there is still less likelihood of infection for single women than for men. Similarly, social conventions restrict the use of alcohol by single girls more than by married women.[3] Apart from these two exceptions, there are no significant sex differences.

Table 21 Marital status and mental disorder, New York (1929–31)

	No. of Cases	*Rate per 100,000 population*
Unmarried	10,473	111·3
Married	12,817	77·7
Widowed	4,387	203·1
Divorced	443	280·1

Up to now we have interpreted the American data as evidence of sociological influences. But can these statistics not be interpreted otherwise? It is easy to reverse the terms of the explanation without destroying the relationship between marital status and mental disorder. If there is more psychosis among unmarried than among married people, this may simply be because the mentally ill do not find marriage partners or tend to shy away from marriage.[4] If the highest percentage is shown by divorced people, this may be because mental disorder becomes manifest while the couple is living together, thus disrupting marital harmony or preventing the sick person from adjusting to married life. Divorcees are people who have had difficulties in relating to each other: they must therefore also be the most unstable people. Finally, for widowed women it is difficult to choose between two explanations, the influence of the family factor (the severing of emotional ties by death) and the influence of the economic factor (financial difficulties caused by the loss of the breadwinner). In spite of these doubts, it remains a fact that unmarried men have twelve times more alcoholic psychosis and syphilitic psychosis than married men, that widowers also show very high rates of alcoholic psychosis and divorcees of paresis and alcoholic psychosis. These are signs that the family does have a stabilizing effect and is an important factor in the achievement and maintenance of mental health. The queries we have just raised do, of course, limit the aetiological interpretation, but they do not destroy it altogether.

A second group of studies is concerned with the child in the family, it does examine the influence of the family as an institution institutional and the interrelational approach to the study of the family, it does, examine the influence of the family as an institution on the mental health of children.

Let us first of all look at family size. According to some sociologists, children who have brothers or sisters are better equipped for life than only children; they learn at an early age how to get along with others; they discover the virtue of adjusting to each other's personalities and of giving in occasionally. Other authors, however, point out that when the family is large parents cannot give their children adequate attention and tend also to have favourites; that children need to develop in an affectionate atmosphere and become aggressive if they are brought up in a climate of jealousy, distrust and rivalry. Wahl, who studied the family background of 392 schizophrenics, found that many of his subjects were from families of four or more children. He also found that the type of schizophrenia varies in relation to the number of children, from simple schizophrenia (3·2 children per family) to the more complicated forms with hebephrenia at the top (4·9 children per family). He suggests that hebephrenia is the expression of a desire to return to childhood.[5] Sanua criticized these conclusions, and pointed out that 34 per cent of the patients studied by Wahl were from Catholic families, which are more prolific, especially in the lower social classes, than Protestant families. If Wahl had used a control group he would probably have found that family sizes were similar in the normal and in the schizophrenic group. As for the proportion of male to female children in the family, Sanua found that in his Jewish sample 30 per cent of the schizophrenic girls were from families composed only of girls. This high percentage is possibly due to the fact that the Jews, with their patriarchal family system, have a stronger desire to have boys: the girls would then feel that they were neither wanted nor loved, but merely tolerated.[6]

While the family unit, whether large or small, appears to be an environment favourable to mental health, the effects of family disruption (by the death of a parent, desertion, separation or divorce) must surely be as pathogenic for the children as they are for the parents. We mentioned earlier Hollingshead and Redlich's study of broken homes in Class V of their social scale (the lowest class), and we regretted that they had not taken this factor into account in their interpretation: 41 per cent of the children under seventeen in this class came from broken homes, and the number of schizophrenics in particular was eight times as high as in Classes I and II combined. Again, Sanua voices doubts about the influence of family disruption on mental disorder. In his sample from the Elgin State Hospital, Wahl found that 43 per cent of the patients had lost one or both parents through death, separation or divorce; however, Sanua points out that other variables must be taken into account, such as sex, social class and religion, as well as the type of schizophrenia: 51 per cent of the Protestant paranoid schizophrenics from the lower class were from broken homes, compared with only 13 per cent of the Jewish paranoid patients. In fact, paranoid schizophrenia tended to be more frequent than catatonic schizophrenia (twice as frequent for all groups taken together). As for sex we find important differences according to ethnic groups and religion. There were more mentally-ill women among the Jews (17 per cent of the female patients were Jewish, as compared with 10 per cent of the men); both sexes were equally represented among the Protestants: 51 per cent of the male patients and 50 per cent of the female patients in the paranoid schizophrenic group were Protestants. Within the same sex and the same religion there were differences according to ethnic group: 41 per cent of the Irish patients were paranoid, as compared with only 11 per cent of the Italian patients. In the second place, Sanua maintains that it is necessary to use a control group: for example, Fisher reckoned that 6·3 per cent of the total population of the U.S.A. had lost one or both parents by the age of eighteen; if we reflect that loss of parents in the Jewish sample amounts only to 10 per cent and that it includes separation and divorce, it appears that, at least for the Jewish group, loss of parents is not a significant variable.

Present-day research tends to concentrate more on neurosis than on psychosis. The findings on neurosis are as follows:

(1) The correlation between neurosis and loss of parents due to death is not significant, but separation or divorce and the presence of mental disorder in the parents do have an effect on very young children, which is manifested later by personality disturbances.

(2) When the mother comes from a broken home or has a disturbed early history, she possesses neurotic tendencies which skip a generation, remaining latent in the mother and breaking out in her child. On the other hand, the father who comes from a broken home and whose childhood was unhappy will do all he can to protect the child from suffering, and thus gives him every chance of good mental health.[7]

(3) One of the most important factors is the existence of a harmonious relationship between the parents. Duhrsen's statistics are very clear on this point. Other authors also show that, where the parents' relations are not satisfactory, it is better for the child that they separate or divorce rather than continue to resent each other and fight in front of their offspring.[8]

(4) The external problems faced by the family, its struggle to make ends meet and its desire to improve the status of its members can have a considerable effect on the offspring. This is especially true if the parents are obliged to leave the child with its grandparents so that it feels it is being abandoned, or if an ambitious father who cannot rise in life himself satisfies his ambitions vicariously through his sons.

(5) Religious ideologies (in particular, those of minority sects) and mixed marriages (between Catholics and Protestants, where the parents fight over the child) can also have pathogenic influences, as Duhrsen pointed out. Mixed marriage has a direct effect, but religious ideologies are more of an indication of the parents' neurotic character, so that we are dealing here, not with the direct influence of the religious culture, but with the transmission of neurotic tendencies expressed in religious behaviour.[9]

From studies of the family background of defective children, it appears that there is a strong tendency for children of unmarried mothers who have been abandoned to show arrested development, both intellectual and emotional. To a certain extent this is also true for children who have been 'half-abandoned' to grandparents or institutions when their parents separate,[10] although the effect is less marked if the child finds a substitute home.

We may therefore conclude that a harmonious family background is necessary to the psychological well-being of the child, and that any disturbance he shows, either during childhood or in later life, is due to a large extent to conflict between the parents. The doubts held by psychiatrists about the effect of broken homes do not invalidate this conclusion. First of all, these doubts apply to psychosis only, and particularly to schizophrenia; the whole range of psychopathology has to be considered if a valid judgment is to be made. Secondly, we have shown that it is better for the mental health of the child for his parents to separate than to stay together and expose him to their incessant hostility and recriminations.

After these general considerations on the psychiatry of the family, we shall now deal at greater length with two particular factors which have attracted the attention of many sociologists and psychiatrists and have produced some interesting research: bereavement and the ordinal position of the child in the family.

Bereavement. Mourning is regulated by cultural norms, which is why this subject more than others has brought about a fruitful collaboration between anthropologists, sociologists and psychiatrists. However, in addition to the culturally determined tie that structures the relationship between husband and wife, and the ritual surrounding the loss of one partner, we must also consider the psychological, affective and intimate bond between husband and wife. Cultural norms can intensify or lessen this emotional bond; to understand the effect of bereavement, it must therefore be studied in its dual context, both interrelational and cultural: in terms of 'the self and its relations with others' and in terms of the 'roles' prescribed by the civilization, which have to be assumed for a conventional period of time.[11] First of all, what are the norms of Western culture? Stroetzel emphasizes the three following features:

(1) Our family is a nuclear family, with few members, where husband and wife normally have a very close emotional tie, and where each partner has a specific role. Consequently, the partner who dies becomes 'irreplaceable'.

(2) In a small family, although there are emotional satisfactions, daily life together is bound to give rise to feelings of hostility, which are probably quickly repressed, but which leave the survivor with anxiety-producing guilt, another possible cause of psychological disturbance.

(3) The role of the mourner is a difficult one: certain behaviour is expected for him which he has not learnt and for which he is therefore unprepared. What is more, the less culturally defined these roles are (at present they are becoming less and less defined), the more at a loss the person feels and the more he risks encountering psychological problems which are injurious in the long run to his mental health.[12]

Let us now view bereavement in terms of the break in affective ties and the personality changes occurring in the survivors. An emotional unit is broken, leaving the survivor in a state of distress; death disrupts a whole series of habits which the couple have built up together and shared and whose abrupt disappearance intensifies the feeling of a gap that cannot be filled. Eliot listed the possible effects of this crisis, which is obviously not merely a psychological crisis, but also a sociological one. The immediate effects are a feeling of being forsaken, refusal to accept death to the extent of perceiving the events as unreal, a reaction of calm, neurosis, exaltation, self-destructive attacks (which can go as far as suicidal attempts), repression of grief, feelings of guilt (the patient blames himself for the death of the loved one or feels that he has not done all he could) and resentment towards others (doctors or other members of the family). Secondary reactions are alcoholism, suicide and other escapist solutions, compensatory rituals (such as perpetuating the memory of the deceased through a sort of cult of the dead), masochism and exhibitionism (seclusion or refusal to see anyone), identification (the survivor reincarnates the dead person or perpetuates him by becoming identified with him) and transference and substitution (the bereaved person shifts his affection to another member of the family). Clearly some of the consequences of bereavement are pathological and others normal according to our culture. If the survivor fails in readjusting to life without his partner, this can produce psychosis (suicide, unconscious death-wish or insanity). If the failure is not total, we merely have neurotic reactions (collapse, lack of motivation, loss of the will to live, seclusion, resentment or self-hate).[13]

These studies help us to understand the importance that loss of spouse assumes in the figures given at the beginning of this chapter. The picture is particularly striking for the older age-groups, as shown by a study made in New York in 1950 on adjustment among the aged:

Table 22   Percentages represented by each marital status group in a sample of mentally-ill old people

Married men, 17·9	Widowers, 28·8
Married women, 17·8	Widows, 27·9
Both groups, 17·9	Both groups, 28·1
Separated and divorced men, 36·6	Unmarried men, 26·0
Separated and divorced women, 29·4	Unmarried women, 24·1
Both groups, 33·3	Both groups, 25·0

However, if one also considers age and economic situation (the death of one of the partners can diminish the resources of the family unit), the difference in the rate of mental disorder between widows and married people is no longer statistically significant. The sole exception to this is the group of men and women aged from sixty-five to seventy-four of low economic status and good physical health.[14]

Birth order. Psychoanalysts have stressed the importance of ordinal position among siblings in the formation of the personality: they have observed psychological differences between first-born, middle and last-born children. The question that can be asked is whether this differentiation is not equally relevant to psychopathology. For example, Wahl found that schizophrenia, both in its paranoid and catatonic forms, was predominant among children of low birth rank.[15] Schooler, who studied a group of female hospitalized schizophrenics, also found that a greater number of patients were born in the lower half of the sibling hierarchy than in the top half. But here many more of them were catatonic than paranoid.[16] Sanua's findings are similar: schizophrenia is found more often among only children and last-born children. In these two ordinal positions catatonic schizophrenia is more frequent than paranoid schizophrenia; Sanua explains this by the fact that mothers tend to show a domineering type of affection for the only or youngest child, thus hampering his normal development.

Table 23 Ordinal position in family and type of schizophrenia

	Paranoid, %	*Catatonic, %*
Only child	14	21
Last-born child	35	43·5
First-born child	35	21·5
Intermediary children	16·5	14[17]

Malzberg made a thorough study of this problem, using various statistical methods. His starting-point is the current assumption that the first-born is more prone to mental disorder than other siblings, as would seem to be the case according to data collected by Heren in a hospital in Perth. (See Table 24.)

However, he is under the impression that many of these first-born children were mentally defective or epileptic and not psychotic at all in the medical sense. He therefore chose a genuine psychosis, dementia praecox, and collected a sample of 549 patients in New York State. He compared the size of these patients' families with the family size for the total population according to the 1930 Census and obtained the figures shown in Table 25.

But the larger the family the more chance that it will have disturbed members. So the data have to be submitted to a special statistical process to correct this error and to obtain the true proportion of first-born children in the psychotic group. By eliminating the single-child families, where the patient is inevitably the first-born (according to the method used by Weinberg, Greenwood and Yule), the following type of result is obtained for a three-child family, the expected percentage represented by the first-born is 17·3 and the observed percentage 16, etc. The method is different, but we reach the same conclusion as previously: the first-born child has an advantage over the other children from the point of view of mental health.[18]

Table 24   Ordinal position and mental disorder in Perth survey

	Per 1,000 patients	Per 1,000 patients in the family stock
First-born	230·8	167·5
Second-born	170·9	159·5
Third-born	166·7	150·4
Fourth-born	151·7	129·6
Fifth-born	87·6	112·4
Sixth-born	70·5	86·6, etc.

Table 25   Ordinal position and dementia praecox

	Census return, %	Dementia praecox, %
1 child	33·2	4·9
2 children	28·8	13·3
3 children	18·0	17·3
4 children	10·0	12·6
5 children	5·1	12·2
6 children	2·5	11·8

A study by Mauco and Rambaud in France came to the opposite conclusion. However, in this case, the subjects were children referred to a psychiatrist for emotional and behaviour problems:

Table 26 Ordinal position and mental disorder

	Clinical cases, %	Census returns,% (per 100 children under twenty-one years)
Only children	33	18
First-born	27	21
Intermediary	20	51
Last-born	19	51

Does this mean that the pattern we found for psychotics is reversed for problem children? Or must we attribute this contradiction (with the exception of only children) to cultural differences between American and French parents which affect their relations with their children according to birth rank? Mauco and Rambaud explain the figures for only children by maternal possessiveness (the only child is weaned later and shares his parents' bedroom two or three times more often than children in larger families). Eldest children, on the other hand, feel displaced by the birth of a sibling after having been the centre of the mother's attention; they also tend to be treated like adults too early (high proportion of Oedipus complexes and sibling jealousy).[19] In intermediary and youngest children the important features are a desire to catch up with the older ones and to gain the attention of adults and a reaction against being called the 'little ones'. There appears to be a progressive decrease, from the first to the last category, in the violence of the traumas experienced, along with a parallel decrease in emotional and personality disorders. The symptoms range from disciplinary problems at school in the only children to instability in the eldest, speech disorders in intermediary children and nervousness in the youngest.[20]

We shall have to wait until other French studies are produced before knowing whether the pattern according to birth order is any different for psychosis and whether the data collected in French hospitals bear any relation to the American data. It is important to note that Mauco and Rambaud's subjects were all under twenty-one, while the American figures are based on the family structure of adult psychotics.

With these last studies we have been led imperceptibly, through the interpretation of the data, from the family as a social institution to the family as a set of interrelations. This will be our approach in the second part of our psychiatric study of the family.

2 The psychiatry of the family from the interrelational viewpoint

There are some studies available on marital relations and their pathology.[21] But under the influence of psychoanalysis, and owing to the particular character of American sociology, which is a sociology of interpersonal relations, psychiatric research has mainly concentrated on the parent-child relationship. We shall therefore confine ourselves to this field.

Psychoanalytic sociology, which is based on Freudian assumptions, has been concerned to show that the individual's fate is sealed in the first few years of life. It maintains that each culture has its particular way of bringing up children and that, according to whether the frustrations of the child are predominantly oral, anal or genital, there will be different adult forms of psychological disturbance.[22] However, within our own civilization there are differences in culture between social classes. In particular, it has been noted that the lower class is much more permissive and the middle class more puritanical; the frustrations experienced by lower-class children tend to be oral, due to a low standard of living, and those of the middle class anal, due to the middle-class emphasis on cleanliness.[23] As we saw in our chapter on ecology, these differences are reflected in the mental disorder patterns of the two groups. These interpretations can be frankly psychoanalytic in character; they then deal with the stages of development of the libido, the causes of its fixations in a particular family setting, or of its regression; they try to discover whether the Oedipus complex is more difficult to resolve in some social classes than in others, etc. Or else they can be more sociologically oriented, as with Erich Fromm: parental restrictions are experienced by the child as commands rather than as sexual conflicts, even of an unconscious nature.[24] Finally, they can consider, as Ruth Benedict did, the continuities and discontinuities between childhood and adolescence, the contrast in Western civilization between the exaggerated protection given to the child and the freedom enjoyed by the adolescent, between sexual taboos during the first years of life and the later glorification of sexual virility.[25]

Clearly, even if these considerations are valid, they cannot contribute much to a sociology of mental disorder, since they merely explain tendencies to develop a particular form of mental pathology. But are they valid explanations even in this context? A comparison of two studies of class differences in child care, one made in Chicago and the other at Harvard, showed that although there were certain common features, the difference between the two communities was considerable. It is therefore dangerous to generalize from a limited sample to a whole class on a national scale; regional or religious factors or the ethnic composition of the population introduce variables which have to be controlled. It is of interest to note in passing that in the study mentioned some of the findings common to both surveys contradict the conclusions mentioned above. The lower class appeared to be stricter and more punitive in toilet-training matters, while the middle-class children enjoyed more freedom of movement out of doors during the day than the lower-class children.[26] But above all we must realize that there is a gap between the sort of upbringing the child receives, which is a 'constant', and mental disorder, which fortunately only appears in a few families. The important thing is not the set of general norms of a particular social class, but the idiosyncratic family conditions in which a child is raised. In short, the method we should follow is not to take social background as a starting-point from which to understand the formation of neurosis or psychosis, but, on the contrary, to start from the phenomena of neurosis and psychosis and work backwards to the structure of family relations which may have produced these disturbances.

Cameron pointed out that obsessional neurosis develops in families that are particularly tyrannical towards the child: when the child grows up he finds himself torn between his past submissive role and the role of the harsh parent whom he has internalized: 'He is alternating in his own self-reaction between the culturally defined social role of the hypercritical, vindictive, domineering parent and the reciprocal social role of the anxious, guilty, penitent child.'[27]

The most penetrating studies which have been made are concerned with the social background of schizophrenics.[28] Attention is mainly centred on the mother, because she is the principal figure in the child's early life: she is found to be either over-protective or aggressive, domineering and rejecting, and the term 'schizophreno-genic mother' has been suggested.[29] Kohn and Clausen took both parents into account: the presence of an authoritarian and castrating mother is one of the conditions for producing schizophrenia; but also the father must be self-effacing, submissive, indifferent or neglecting (so that he cannot be internalized by the child in the form of a superego).[30] On the other hand, most of the patients studied by Helen Frazee had strict, cruel and rejecting fathers.

165

As she points out, this finding is interesting because it goes against the general assumption of psychiatric literature that the father tends to be passive and ineffectual.[31] As for the French studies, Sivadon, Mises and Mises think that the domineering mother is the main factor in the causation of schizophrenia,[32] while other authors think that an ineffectual or passive father is a much more important factor.[33]

But might these contradictions not disappear if, instead of looking at schizophrenia in general, we broke it down into various types? According to Arieti:

> The mother of the paranoid patient does not criticize her child for his actions, but accuses him of bad intentions. . . . This develops in the child a facility for rationalization which enables him to protect himself from insinuations and accusations. . . . The catatonic patient, on the other hand, has never been able to develop a capacity to decide anything for himself because the parents impose their own will on him as a child. The catatonic defence represents a struggle between the incorporated image of the parents and the patient's own wishes, a conflict that seems to resolve itself by complete inactivity.[34]

On the basis of these hypotheses we may conclude that paranoid schizophrenia occurs primarily in families where the child is rejected by his parents, and that catatonic schizophrenia tends to occur in over-protective families. Hitson and Funkestein, who compared paranoid schizophrenia in two widely different cultures, those of Boston and Burma, emphasized the importance of 'social distance' in communication between parents and children. To confine ourselves to Boston, since we are excluding ethnopsychiatry from this book, it appears that the father in the families of paranoid schizophrenics is the sole source of authority, and the mother the sole source of affection. The child realizes that it is impossible for him to have any control over his social environment, and that his actions seem unpredictable to the people around him. Faced with his father's condemnations and his mother's distress, he reacts by justifying his actions in his own eyes, by making up stories, rationalizing what are essentially spontaneous actions, and thus developing paranoid tendencies. On the other hand, patients suffering from depression tend to have parents who have always satisfied their wishes; the child becomes an object manipulated by others to maintain a peaceful and happy atmosphere in the family. Later, however, the pampered and over-protected child soon comes to the realization that other people are indifferent to his desires and ambitions and that society is not one big, protective family. Hence his attacks of depression.[35] These findings show a similarity to Arieti's: rejection on the one hand and over-protection on the other. The empirical research done by Sanua, which we mentioned previously in relation to religious groups, confirms that parental rejection is two to three times as frequent in the families of paranoid patients as in the families of catatonics.[36]

Thus the disagreement between psychiatrists is mainly due to the fact that they do not take into account the various types of schizophrenia. Wahl maintains that schizophrenia is caused by rejection, but this is in fact because only 15 per cent of his sample are catatonics; the part played by over-protection is therefore masked. Others, on the contrary, such as Gérard and Siegel, consider over-protection to be the dominant factor, but this is merely because about 50 per cent of their sample are catatonics.[37] The predominant family type naturally differs according to social class, ethnic group and religious group, which would account for particular sociological variations; however, each one of these groups includes parents who spoil their children and others who reject them, and therefore both catatonic and paranoid schizophrenics.

Psychoanalytic sociology in the U.S.A. has been undergoing a crisis in the past few years. Its critics (Lindesmith and Strauss, for example,[38] or Sewell[39]) mainly object to the over-emphasis on the effect of oral and anal frustration on the mental health of the individual. In his study of 162 American farm children, Sewell found that adaptability to new circumstances did not vary according to the type of training experienced. Breast-fed children were no different from bottle-fed ones, children weaned gradually from those weaned abruptly, and children punished for accidents during toilet-training from those who were not. The only significant factor was the age at which the children experienced anal frustration. Similarly, for rejection and over-protection, Sewell did not find any significant differences between children who were very much attached to their mother and children who were not, and between those who lived in an atmosphere of emotional security and those who did not. Nevertheless, he does not conclude that childhood is an unimportant period for determining future psychological equilibrium, but maintains that the crucial factor is not the way feeding and toilet-training are practised, but the total situation in which they occur and particularly the attitudes and behaviour of the mother. Such research as Arieti's is thus able to survive the criticism prevalent today, particularly in the 'culture and personality' school, who are increasingly concerned with minimizing the importance of parental practices.

There are many other studies, empirical or clinical, statistical or interpretative, which we could have reported in each of the previous chapters; we have confined ourselves to quoting and summarizing those which seem the most significant.

We can now return to the issues we raised at the beginning of ch. III and which we left in abeyance. So far we have confined ourselves to contrasting the different theories while reserving the final answer until we had reviewed all the social factors that have been considered aetiologically significant. The issue is whether sociogenesis is applicable both to so-called reactive psychosis and to neurosis.

IX The ordering of the material

The reader who has followed us through this confusion of studies on mental illness in various groups may well by now be feeling discouraged. It is as if we were dealing with a jig-saw puzzle with many missing pieces which have been replaced by bits from other puzzles: parts of the picture do not fit in, shapes refuse to interlock. We can try to reconstruct the picture, albeit with gaps, but the only thing we succeed in doing, since the bits come from different puzzles, is to create an ordered chaos.

The total number of hospitalized patients is sometimes given in census returns, but these total figures cannot provide us with a starting-point for a sociology of mental disorder: the different variables have to be controlled and we therefore need to select a smaller sample. We have seen in the previous chapters how psychiatrists and sociologists, often working together, have tried to refine their statistical methods and supplement their quantitative studies by case histories. But inevitably what their research has gained in precision it has lost in comprehensiveness. Some excellent studies have been made of patients in particular mental hospitals. But how can this micro-sociology help us to reach the macro-sociological view which is our aim? It is as if we were gazing at a sky filled with stars: some are brighter than others, but when viewed all together they still do not make up the Milky Way we are searching for.

The findings of these fragmentary studies are difficult to compare and cannot easily be used to complete each other. The techniques they employ are different, and it is well known that the method of a study is part of its aim; in other words, that recorded data are not so much facts as mental constructions. We are again faced with our metaphor of the mixed-up pieces of puzzle. Objects constructed with different techniques cannot be compared: they belong to different methodological realms. We should therefore not be surprised if we find that the results of various studies, instead of confirming each other, tend to be in contradiction. However, let us accept, in spite of our previous criticism, that this type of research does provide objective findings. From the point of view of the sociology of mental disorder, these studies, then, contain, when we try to compare them, an internal contradiction. Each geographical region has its own culture or, to be more precise, its own subculture: social structures present the most remarkable contradictions; ecological differences are too obvious to be missed. If we make the assumption of our own particular branch of sociology that mental disturbance expresses the influence of culture, environment and social organization, then we shall never be able to make comparisons between, for example, the patients of a small town in the Southern States of America and those in a neighbourhood of New York City. We are trapped in the particular and are unable to discover general laws. Another serious handicap is that there are different schools of psychiatry: diagnosis follows academic traditions, the classification of psychosis varies from school to school. The author came up against this difficulty in his work in Brazil. He found that for out-patients, depending on which doctor made the diagnosis, the proportion of different types of psychosis varied and the actual ratio of neurosis to psychosis was altered. Such are the studies we are dealing with that we are not even sure of the reliability of the data we wish to compare.

1 Sociocultural factors

It is necessary to pause for a while and to take a step back from this confusion of heterogeneous studies. Now that we have collected them all together, perhaps we can come to a few conclusions about the importance of sociocultural factors in the aetiology of mental illness.

Let us start with the simpler question of neurosis. Here we find two theories: neurosis can be interpreted with reference either to the sociology of the family or to the sociology of Western society. What produces neurosis? Is it the relationship children have with their parents and the way their basic training is given by their mother or father? Or is neurosis created by the contradictions of capitalist society, the confusion and difficulties of city life, the ever-increasing variety and the often contradictory nature of the roles the individual is expected to play? We mentioned more than once that this is the conflict between the supporters of traditional psycho-analysis and the Neo-Freudians. There has sometimes been an attempt, as with Sullivan and his followers, to transcend the debate and reconcile the data from various sources by stating that early experience may be important, but that the individual's fate should not be considered sealed in infancy. Every person evolves and changes and it is not only childhood experience that is important, but also the experience of the adolescent, who is often thrown into a world for which he is ill-prepared and which, by this simple fact, can be traumatic. The psychoanalyst's approach is to try to work back into the distant past of the neurotic patient; the psychiatrist, on the other hand, tries to reconstruct the whole of the patient's life history, both emotional and intellectual, without putting any more emphasis on one period than on another. It would be feasible to develop a sociology of neurosis based on this synthetic approach by listing the successive social traumas the individual experiences from his childhood onwards.[1]

Ruth Benedict's idea of cultural 'continuities' and 'discontinuities'[2] can help us to understand how the greater social environment can have an effect, in addition to the earlier influence of the family. Her approach is better than the synthetic approach, which is inevitably eclectic; it is a genuine theory. When there is no discontinuity between what is expected of the child and what is expected of the adult, as in many primitive societies, neurosis does not appear. However, in Western society, radically different behaviour is required of different age-groups. The child is protected and at the same time restricted, while the man is expected to show initiative, enterprise and sexual virility. When the individual passes from one age-group to another he finds that the roles which used to be prohibited now become compulsory; he has to graduate from irresponsibility to responsibility, from submissiveness to freedom of action and even to authority over others when he becomes a father or holds a position of power in the occupational world, from sexual abstinence to the full expression of his virility. These cultural discontinuities are characteristic of our society. Maladjustment is the result of the individual remaining fixated at a pre-adult level, unable to take the step—the plunge, in fact—that our civilization expects of him. If we accept this point of view, it becomes easier to see how neurosis can be determined both by famly influences and by the discontinuous structures of society. When Karen Horney, whose theories we outlined earlier, speaks of the 'neurosis of our time', she is only describing the internalization in the individual consciousness of the conflicts between the requirements of different stages of human life.

Without rejecting orthodox Freudian theory, we can still recognize the importance of contemporaneous social factors in the causation of neurosis. There has been too much emphasis on the aspect of Freud's work concerned with the fixation of the libido at infantile stages, to the detriment of another aspect of his theory. Neurosis is not produced by infantile traumas, but by the meeting of an old and a new trauma; for neurosis to occur it is not sufficient for there to have been a shock in early childhood: this shock has to be reactivated by the social situation of the adult. This provides us with an aetiological model with two entries, where both 'micro'- and 'macro'-sociology can coexist: a theory developed on this basis would be a theory of recurrence. We can do no more here than to sketch its main outlines. All social structures present formal analogies in the shape of conflicts, discrepancies and internal contradictions. They expect of the individual particular behaviour patterns which can be classified into various reactive types. When society presents to the individual a situation similar to the one that was traumatic for him in early childhood and expects him to behave in the way he did then, neurosis appears. Thus loss of spouse can reawaken the situation of maternal deprivation, and the experience of dealing with a rigid bureaucratic organization can recall painful episodes with a strict father. Here again the combination of family influences and social influences is more than a simple addition of factors; both types of influence are integrated into an organic whole.

The reader may accuse us at this stage of leaving out constitutional factors; we have spoken of external 'triggers' to neurosis while appearing to ignore the 'host'. A valid aetiology must surely recognize that there is such a thing as a 'predisposed' individual. Our theory must therefore be completed by introducing this third dimension. Personally, we accept Pierre Janet's idea, which we mentioned in our historical introduction, of psychic energy or 'tension' (which would correspond to nervous or cerebral energy). We also accept Vie's idea of psychic 'thresholds': society expects us to perform increasingly complicated tasks, and individuals who do not have the necessary energy will have a low threshold in terms of performance of the required activities.

> We tried to show how the simple activity of digestion differs from the activity of dining out, dressed in a dinner-jacket, in the company of a lady. Similarly, sexual activities have a very simple and primitive basis, but they have been infinitely complicated by the addition first of social tendencies, then of intellectual activities in the form of reflection about possible consequences, then of tendencies to moral criticism, etc. This is why there can so easily be disorders associated with dining out, and why there is a whole psychopathology of the engagement and the honeymoon. . . . When a person is led to think about an activity, to give it a social or ethical significance, he renders the activity much more difficult; he

makes it into a reality and draws upon more recently
developed tendencies. This process becomes obvious in the
pathology of professional and religious activities. Conversely,
it is possible, by various artifices, to make these activities
easier. It is often less difficult to perform an activity for another
person than for ourselves, because it is of less importance to
us; it is easier to perform an activity secretly than in public;
finally, it is interesting to note that when an activity is left
until the appropriate moment is over, the later it is performed
the easier it becomes.[3]

We may admit that there are 'strong' and 'weak' constitutions; it
is nevertheless true that certain family backgrounds can render a
strong subject more vulnerable. Early training can raise or lower
the threshold of resistance of the psyche to the difficulties encountered in adult life. Thus 'predisposition' has both a constitutional and a sociological basis. We cannot separate the elements of
the *Gestalt*. In fact, *Gestalt* is probably the most appropriate term
to use for a model where the various components, personal, familial
and social, are mutually dependent and form a single system of
interrelations which must always be grasped in its organic totality.

We have left aside the question of therapy, as this is the particular
field of the psychiatrist. However, therapy provides a sort of double
check in the verification of our hypothesis and, at least in that
particular capacity, it cannot be entirely ignored. Therapy is a
purposeful manipulation of pathological phenomena. It therefore
constitutes a planned experiment just as social planning, on the
level of society as a whole, is a substitute for sociological experimentation. Previously we examined the characteristics of Soviet
psychiatry. Its first premise is that there is a difference in nature
between the psychoses, which are explained by the mental or
biological constitution of the individual, and the neuroses, which
are the outcome of conditioned responses or of their inhibition, but
which in the last analysis are sociological phenomena, since they
are conditioned by social groups. It also maintains that neurosis is a
product of the contradictions of the class-system and as such must
disappear along with social classes. What has happened in reality?
Neurosis has indeed disappeared from the statistics, but it is now
found in general hospitals in the form of somatic disturbance.
Even if we do not accept the statement of the opponents of communism that the old class system in Russia has been replaced by
a new one (the bureaucratic class instead of the former ruling class),
even if we take the communist ideological standpoint that social
classes have indeed disappeared, we must not forget that communist
ideology recognizes the existence of contradictions between occu-

173

pational categories. As we stated earlier, what is important is not the similarity of content, but the similarity of structural forms. The manipulation of neurosis in Soviet Russia confirms two of our hypotheses. First, individual predisposition must be taken into account (neurosis has not disappeared along with the class struggle), whether this predisposition is constitutional or the outcome of the family situation. Second, the greater social environment plays a part; it intervenes in this instance by exerting pressure to orient disturbances along somatic lines rather than along lines which might be contrary to Marxist-Leninist doctrine.

If we now compare Soviet with Western psychiatry, we find that the latter consists of a reorganization of the personality, a transformation of a fragmented and damaged ego into a richer and more unified one. Rogers, in recording the various phases of treatment, noticed that the neurotic patient, or 'sick ego', carries within him a number of elements which have not been experienced because of their association with parental restrictions in the early stages of training. These elements have acquired a 'negative valence'; they have been repressed, and thus constitute a threatening zone in the individual's self-perception. Psychotherapy enables the subject to experience these elements: it is a re-education of the patient and therefore a social phenomenon.[4]

We now need to see whether the statements we have made for neurosis are also valid for psychosis.

If the number of psychotics were growing faster than the world population, it could be inferred that social influences are more important than biological ones. If particular mental disorders, such as schizophrenia and paranoia (the two illnesses discussed most by anthropologists), did not exist in every *culture* (we are not saying *race* or *ethnic group*), the sociology of mental disorder would indeed become an aetiology. If, on the other hand, statistics were to show that, in spite of changes in social structure and differences between cultures, the incidence of psychosis remains constant, then the sociology of mental disorder would no longer offer a valid or complete explanation of mental disorder. According to Clausen, cultural conflicts and feelings of frustration can lead to behaviour disorders, but there is no evidence that they lead to psychosis.

In fact, the statistics are not conclusive in either direction. However, we shall deliberately adopt the hypothesis furthest removed from the sociological explanation. Even in this case it is an obvious fact that psychosis tends to be concentrated in particular sectors of society. Some areas are pathogenic. This localization of mental disorder may not allow us to evolve an explanatory theory, but it does provide a basis for mental-health policies. The problem is the same as for crime, where there is also a heated discussion about the relative importance of constitutional and social factors. Even though the issue is not yet settled, the distribution of crime in zones has been widely used as a guide for preventive policies, apparently with fruitful results.

Another fact which becomes obvious is that the manifestations of psychosis vary according to the social setting—one could also add: according to the period. American psychiatrists have noticed changes in the nature of schizophrenia over the last thirty or forty years: regressive symptoms have disappeared, due to the lack of activation of oral and anal factors in contemporary society.[5] Thus if sociology does not provide us with an aetiology, at least it gives us an epidemiology. We may accept the existence of morbid constitutions, but can we now predict the sort of illness towards which they will evolve? The answer is that their outcome is impossible to determine, since it depends entirely on the social situation and on cultural pressures. As we have already noted, the change from latent to manifest morbidity follows particular avenues determined by the structures of society and by the values and norms of civilization. For example, the research which has been done on the role of the castrating mother or the passive father in the causation of catatonic or paranoid schizophrenia is sufficiently supported by controlled case studies for us to accept the fact that the patient's family background determines whether he will develop catatonic or paranoid symptoms. It is exactly as if our society were training morbid personalities to develop along specific lines and produce particular types of psychosis. This aspect of the problem—the existence of a sociology of the manifestations of mental disorder—would have stood out even more clearly if, instead of remaining within our civilization, we had become ethnologists and extended our survey to other cultures.

However, some years ago such authors as Delmas or Boll suggested the existence of psychological types: the effective type, the mythomaniac type, the cyclical type, etc., mental disorder being the exaggeration or caricature of these normal types. This idea has been heavily criticized recently. It is based on the theories of the early psychologists, of whom Ribot is the most typical representative: he considered that pathological phenomena differed only in degree from normal phenomena and endeavoured to understand the normal in terms of the pathological. Since Canguilhem's criticism of this definition of the pathological, to which we referred in an earlier chapter, this sort of theory is no longer relevant. Moreover, it is based on the existence of rigid psychiatric types, an idea which had its heyday, but was disproved by dynamic psychiatry. But even if we were to accept Delmas's point of view, a sociological approach to the study of mental disorder would still remain meaningful. As we have seen several times—for example, in our analysis of 'reactive' psychosis and of the significance of 'events' for the psychotic, or, again, in our study of the role of migration and mobility—the important thing is not the event in itself, or the migration, but its subjective evaluation by the individual, the way in which the individual experiences the social situation in which he is involved. The social factor is obviously not a 'cause', but a 'justification' or 'rationalization'. We still end up with sociology, although it is of a different kind—the sociology of society as experienced by the mentally ill. (We shall later deal with it at greater length.)

Broadly speaking, either we must postulate the antecedence of an undifferentiated morbid constitution (which seems to us the most sensible hypothesis), in which case the part society plays is to shape it, to orient it towards a particular form of disturbance, or, conversely, we can postulate the existence of differentiated constitutional types (schizoid, syntonic, epileptoid, etc., as Bleuler and Minkowski did[6]), in which case the social environment is experienced and rethought through their mediation. They act, if not as direct stimuli, then at least as particular reflections of the situation. But we now fall into a truism, since it is an obvious fact that society can only operate through the individual psyche. All we are concerned with here is that it does operate.

2   A sociological theory of mental disorder

Thus we have evolved a sociological theory of mental disorder similar to the snowball (or 'cumulative') principle, which was clearly illustrated by Gunnar Myrdal first in the field of economics and later, as we shall see, in relation to the Negro problem.[7] Myrdal replaces the notion of static equilibrium (implicit in the concepts of accommodation, adjustment, maladjustment, etc.) by the idea of a dynamic whole, a system in constant flux, inspired by dynamic economics. He makes wide use of the concept of the vicious circle with reference to the American Negro: the more prejudice there is against the Negro, the worse his social situation becomes; reciprocally, prejudice against him increases the more his way of life sinks below that of the whites. There is a mutual interaction between these two variables, and the cumulative process which results means that we can no longer speak in terms of mechanical causality nor present a simple explanatory model. A change in one of the forces acting on the system (even if it is in a different direction from the other forces) is swept along in the cumulative effect of a total system in motion. In short, causal relationships cannot be conveyed by an abstract representation which renders static what is in reality in perpetual transformation. In our opinion, the system Myrdal evolved in his study of the American dilemma, dynamic social causality, can also be applied to a theory of psychosis: psychosis shows the same circular process between the individual and society as that which Myrdal found between the standard of living of the Negro and racial prejudice. We need only to dynamize—if the reader will accept this neologism —the static theory advanced by Delmas to be able to see, for the first time since the beginning of this section on psychosis and just when we seemed furthest removed from a sociological conception of the aetiology of mental disorder, the social factor as a causative factor and not only as a semiological factor.

We must beware of the fallacy of basing the interpretation of human phenomena on mechanical models. The mechanical model has two aspects which are equally inapplicable to human behaviour. The first is the separation in time of cause and effect, the assumption that there is a 'before' and an 'after' (the morbid constitution or the social influence and the subsequent psychosis). The second aspect belongs to our own field of sociology, where Gurvitch has done much to undermine the mechanical conception of causality.[8] His principle of 'reciprocal perspectives' regards society as situated within the psyche and the individual consciousness, in return, as part and parcel of society. It enables us to replace mechanical causality by a system of parallel or symmetrical perspectives. This gives us a way out of the dilemma we stressed in our chapter on ecology between Faris's interpretation of the concentration of mental disorders in some areas as being due to social disintegration and the breaking-up of interpersonal relations into molecular units and Park's explanation that people who are already sick or have pathogenic predispositions tend to drift towards the zones of social isolation. The trouble with this question is that it is badly stated. The two factors, social disorganization and individual disorganization, are merely two aspects of one and the same reality, the same field viewed from two different but reciprocal perspectives. This reciprocity of perspectives is not the only dialectical process involved. Society and the individual psyche implicate each other mutually to the extent that they can be placed in reciprocal perspective, but they can also be in contradiction; psychiatrists have even tended to emphasize this contradictory aspect, illness being viewed as a break in communication. Gurvitch defines it as 'opposites complementing each other within a whole in a dual movement which consists of growing and intensifying, sometimes in the same direction and sometimes in opposite directions, owing to the mechanism of compensation'.

Let us look back over the preceding chapters and follow this dual movement. We saw, for example, that if there are more psychotics in certain ecological areas, that is because of differences in types of residence. This led us from ecology to the study of social class, ethnic groups (where immigrants are concerned) and religion. In pursuing our research further, we found that these sociological variables only took effect through the mode of upbringing received in the family, the relations between parents and children, and the ordinal position of the child. However, at the same time we noted that the privileges of a particular ordinal position were determined by the value-system of society as a whole, that upbringing varied according to social class (working, middle or upper), ethnic group (patriarchal or egalitarian) and religion (puritanical or permissive). We became caught up in two different circuits, apparently in contradiction, which tossed us, like the ebb and flow of the wave, from the general to the particular and back again. This is where Myrdal's principle takes on its full methodological significance and where we can see the relevance of the first part of Gurvitch's phrase: 'which consists of growing and intensifying in the same direction'. The different variables must not be viewed as a mechanism or a set of isolated factors coming into play separately, adding to each other or subtracting from each other, and eventually behaving according to a 'law of resolution of forces'. They must be grasped in a dynamic way, as a total system in motion where it is impossible to make an analytical separation between the influences of the psychic constitution, micro-groups and macro-groups, to detect a 'before' or an 'after'; everything holds together in mutual dependency. The psyche acts as a 'filter' which only accepts those parts of society which can feed and nurture its psychopathy, or as an echo-chamber which amplifies the traumas of social contacts. Reciprocally, society shapes the morbid personality and provides it with what we earlier described as the oxygen necessary to combustion. There is no zero point from which to build up a chronology of influences, since the future patient is enmeshed from birth in familial interrelations, and these interrelations are decided by the family's position in terms of social class, ethnic membership and religious affiliation.

Let us now follow the second process which Gurvitch's sentence suggests, the movement in 'opposite directions' which culminates in the polarity of sick individual and normal society. As the number of roles we are called upon to play in society increases, as the speed of social and cultural change to which we have to adapt is accelerated and the exploitation of one class by another becomes more threatening, individuals predisposed to mental disorder find themselves in social situations with which they cannot deal. Should we say in this case that heredity and constitution are the 'causes' or that it is the complexity of social life which is responsible or, alternatively, the gap which both psychiatrist and sociologist have noticed between the personality and the environment? To wish at all costs to establish between these two factors acting in opposite directions—the psyche and society—which is the main factor is to return to a mechanistic conception. The personality cannot adjust, both because it is sick and because the social situation is too traumatic; the gap between the two, which is a 'social fact', derives from their mutual implication in a dynamic whole oriented towards a split rather than a culmination. But the process is the same, the dialectic of the same nature, and Myrdal's model is still applicable (although apparently in a contradictory manner).

It might seem that we are not far removed basically from the early social psychiatrists, since they maintained, on the one hand, that sociocultural factors only take effect through heredity and physiology, and, on the other, that social influences come into play to 'trigger off' disturbance and act as an 'opportunity' for illness. But a little thought will show how far we are from this interpretation, which remains in its approach essentially Aristotelian, whereas we are viewing things in terms of systems in motion, oriented variables and fluctuating realities. This new perspective is the only one which allows us to speak in terms of a sociologically-oriented aetiology of mental disorder. In fact these terms may no longer apply, and it might be more appropriate to say 'Madness is a social phenomenon' rather than 'Madness has social causes'.

Before concluding we still need to test our theory both for neurosis and psychosis. We stated that therapy, as a manipulative process, constitutes a genuine experiment. We shall therefore take the aspect of therapy which seems the least related to sociology, so that our test will be as stringent as possible: drug treatment, or what has sometimes been called the 'chemical strait-jacket'. We shall refer here to two theses presented in 1964. The first is by F. Dagonet, *La Raison et les Remèdes*. It points out that drugs merely achieve a suspension of the cruder and more visible manifestations of disturbance, a suppression of 'that in which illness seems to reside' (immoderate behaviour), a dampening or an extinction of reactive aggression, without revealing anything about the disorder: 'There is no such thing as a magic potion that can change a person.' The second thesis, by Michel Niqué, is entitled *La Psychopharmacologie*. It is more illuminating still to our issue, since it is clearly opposed to a mechanistic conception: '[Drug] therapy is only a treatment of symptoms and not of causes.' Niqué demonstrates that the effects of drug therapy are not chemical or mechanical, but psychotherapeutic. It acts as a form of gratification for the patient, or of aggression from the psychiatrist against the patient;

in other words, it is a 'symbolic realization'.[9] In fact, one of the author's conclusions is that if the drug is administered orally, as a bottle is given to a baby, it succeeds only on condition that the therapist takes on the role of mother. Only when a dynamic element is introduced to supplement the static effect of the drug can a favourable evolution take place.[10] If, on the contrary, the relationship takes on a sado-masochistic tone, and if the drug is administered forcibly in an atmosphere of hostility, therapy is bound to fail, because it only makes the sick person retreat further into his own world.

In the final analysis, so-called psychological drug therapy is valuable only if it helps to establish and remodel the sociological relationship between two people. Here again we have our dialectic of mutual complementality confirmed in a sense by this particular test.

> The subject's relationship with others is mediated and expressed by his body; by chemically modifying the 'body-state' the drug modifies the subject's ability to make relationships. However, it also represents an object which is given and received. In this capacity it is a means of modifying the particular situation of the psychotherapeutic relationship, since it mediates, represents and energizes part of the psychotherapeutic experience.[11]

We hope this dynamic approach to the aetiology of mental illness will pave the way to a better understanding between psychiatrists, psychologists and sociologists, and that it will promote the integration of all the branches of sociological research we have summarized and discussed in this book by divorcing them clearly from the study of cerebral dysfunctions. But even if we must cling at all costs to the idea of the primacy of physical over mental and social phenomena, there is still justification for a sociology of mental disorder, since insanity remains essentially a 'social phenomenon', like crime or suicide. Therefore the last remaining task is to carry out a structuralist study of mental disorder. Structuralism is different from the sociological approach which we have adopted so far and which, in spite of the work of some French writers, is primarily American, since it tends to shelve the problem of causes.

Structuralism started with Durkheim. He switched from a 'physical' conception of causality in *Rules of Scientific Method* to a symbolic conception of social reality in *Elementary Forms of the Religious Life*. Society is symbolically expressed in the individual in the form of religious beliefs and practices. This is not to say that religion is the product of society in a simple cause-effect, antecedent-consequent relationship, but that in moments of fervour the collective conscience takes on a religious significance for the individual who participates in it. Thus the idea of symbolism is the pivotal idea of this new sociology.

Mauss goes one step further in a text addressed to psychologists and psychiatrists:

> For a long time now, Durkheim and I have shown that communion and communication between people always takes place through symbols, permanent signs which people have in common; these are external to individual mental states which are simply experienced 'successively'; they represent groups of states which are then taken for realities. We have thought for a long time that one of the characteristics of the social fact is precisely this symbolic aspect. Most collective representations are not a unique representation of a unique object, but a representation chosen arbitrarily or more or less arbitrarily to signify another object and to determine the appropriate behaviour. Now we are confident in the value of our theory by the very fact that we can agree with you.

Later he adds:

> It might seem at first sight that sociology can provide no new psychological or psychophysiological symbolism since *the mental mechanisms of the collective life of the individual are not as such any different from the mechanisms of individual consciousness* [our italics]. But whereas you only come across these cases of symbolism relatively rarely and often in sets of abnormal phenomena, we come across them constantly in large numbers and in vast sets of normal phenomena. In every field of sociology we can harvest great quantities of symbols and lay the produce at your feet.[12]

Thus, when Durkheim confined himself to defining the symbolic character of social life, Mauss suggested how the study of pathological symbolism (to which psychoanalysis had just drawn attention at the time) and sociological symbolism could be brought together. His basic idea was that the symbolization process is the same in both cases and that it is consequently possible to envisage a general theory which would explain equally well—in Mauss's words, 'the important elements of myths, rites and beliefs and of the faith in their efficacy; of illusions, religious and esthetic hallucinations, collective mystifications and delusions and their correctives'.

But how can we integrate two types of symbolism that seem so blatantly opposed, the symbolism of the mentally ill being 'personal' and incommunicable, while the other is collective and forms the basis of communion or at least of community? This is the question

Lévi-Strauss answers when he assumes that these symbols are not contingent phenomena, occurring by chance alone, but that they constitute a structuring of basic mental activity, and that by following certain rules one structure can be transformed into another. In the text we shall now quote, which deals with the cultural activities of man, Lévi-Strauss is conscious of the place which pathological subsystems occupy within the cultural system:

> The ensemble of a people's customs always has its particular style: they form into systems. I am convinced that the number of these systems is not unlimited and that human societies, like individual human beings (at play, in their dreams or in moments of delirium) never create absolutely: all they can do is to choose certain combinations from a repertory of ideas which it should be possible to reconstitute. For this one must make an inventory of all the customs which have been observed by oneself or others, the customs pictured in mythology, and the customs evoked both by children and grown-ups in their games. The dreams of individuals, whether healthy or sick, and psychopathological behaviour should also be taken into account. With all this one could eventually establish a sort of periodical chart of chemical elements analogous to that devised by Mendel. In this all customs, whether real or merely possible, would be grouped by families, and all that would remain for us to do would be to recognize those which societies had, in point of fact, adopted.[13]

This quotation has brought us another step forward. In his speech addressed to psychologists, Mauss still regards symbols as concrete realities (the totem, the flag, etc.). Lévi-Strauss, on the other hand, views things in terms of human activity. He may start with cultural activity, but only to discover that behind it lies symbolic activity *in its broadest sense*, which consists in giving a meaning to objects, in turning objects into significations. What is more important, while classical psychiatrists and psychoanalysts start with the pathological and progress to the normal, here the pathological is integrated with the normal into a total system. It is the rules of this system that are important and not the comparison between abnormality and mental health. If we accept this approach, we find that structuralism is proposing a study of the relative importance, the location and the subsequent interaction of the pathological and the normal in organized structures (which are formal structures, but are nevertheless of the order of sociological formalism).

From this point of view it becomes unnecessary to know whether mental disorder has a physiological origin or not, because what the sociologist is trying to see in mental disorder is the symbolic activity and its location in the total structures of collective symbolic systems. In *Structural Anthropology* Lévi-Strauss gives us a glimpse of the possible triumph of a biochemical explanation of psychosis and neurosis. He concludes that in this instance the pathological would not be beyond the range of sociology; on the contrary, it would become a more integral part of it, since in this case the shamanistic cure and the psychoanalytic cure would become identical, and both would represent an organic transformation induced or expressed by a myth.

But there are other passages in Lévi-Strauss's work that point in the opposite direction. We are no longer, then, dealing with mental structures as a foundation for social structures, but with social structures as such. For example:

A particular society is . . . comparable to a universe where only discrete masses are highly structured. It is therefore inevitable that in every society a percentage (which is in fact variable)[14] of individuals find themselves as it were outside the system, or between two or more irreducible systems. These people are expected and even forced by the group to make certain forms of compromise which cannot be realized on a collective level, to feign imaginary transitions and to embody incompatible syntheses. In all these seemingly aberrant behaviours, the 'mentally sick' are only transcribing a particular state of the group and rendering manifest one of its constants. Their peripheral position with regard to a subsystem does not prevent them from being, as much as the subsystem, part of the total system. In other words, if they did not take on this role of obedient witnesses, the total system would run the risk of disintegrating into its subsystems.[15]

Here again we can see that it is not important to know the origin of the disturbances, whether they are related to the soma, the psyche or social tensions. The point is to situate the mentally ill within the collective, to define their structural position. Lévi-Strauss borrows the example of shamanism from Nadel: the *shaman* may well show pathological traits, but he is nevertheless an element of social equilibrium. Nadel suggests that if a comparative study were made of societies with and without *shamans*, it might well show that under the effect of contact with other civilizations, non-shamanistic societies develop a higher incidence of psychosis and neurosis, while in shamanistic societies there is an increase in shamanism without a parallel increase in mental disorder.[16] This example is perhaps more relevant to ethnopsychiatry than to sociology, but we shall see that Western society exhibits similar phenomena.

183

We now find ourselves at the juncture of two paths, both of which lead towards a sociology of mental disorder free from aetiological considerations. The first is based on the complementality of the symbolic activity of the sane and the insane in the structures of the collective mind. The second is based on the complementality of the sane and the insane in the structures of society as a whole. The two do not necessarily constitute separate realms, but rather two means of approach (as the analogy with paths suggests), if it can be shown that social structures are in fact the actualized expression of mental structures (which seems to be the latest theory of Lévi-Strauss) or if it can be shown that mental structures are the reflection of social structures. (This would be the point of view of a particular Marxism which goes beyond the content of ideologies to examine ideological activity in itself.) What discoveries have already been made that can take us further along these two roads? Which psychiatric and sociological authors can provide the elements to build this structural sociology of mental disorder? How can we co-ordinate these elements and transcend them, if possible, to lay the foundations of a more systematic theory? These are some of the questions we must now attempt to answer.

X Society and the 'insane'

1 Sources of data

There are three main sources of data on the role played by the insane in society. Although they do not exactly fit into the perspective we are adopting in the last part of this book, they are nevertheless worthy of our attention:

(1) Historical studies of the conceptions of mental disorder prevalent at different periods, completed by studies of present-day lay conceptions of psychiatric matters.

(2) Studies of the social relations between doctors and patients and of the psychiatric hospital as a social institution or complex of interrelations between patients, nurses, doctors and administrators.

(3) Studies of the reintegration of 'rehabilitated' patients into society.

We must first briefly summarize the principal conclusions emerging from this body of research before we fit them into our total picture.

Historical studies. It is well known that for the primitive mind insanity is a sacred phenomenon, either religious or demonic. Even in the New Testament madness is considered to be possession by evil spirits which must be exorcized in order for the madman to be cured. With the Greeks, medicine became a science; but whereas for somatic illness it could give rational explanations that were universally accepted, it met with resistance as far as illnesses of the mind were concerned; the latter seemed to evade scientific treatment and remained shrouded in mystical conceptions. The Romans made a very great effort to differentiate between various types of mental disturbance, but they were mainly concerned with the social consequences of madness, the disturbances it produces in the com-

munity, and not with its origin. The advent of Christianity sys-
tematically reinforced the archaic conceptions by providing the
medical men (and the theologians) with a Manichaean system of
delusions and incongruous behaviour seen as the fruits of sin, the
manifestations in man of the struggle between God and Satan for
power over the world. With the Renaissance began what the Americans term 'secularization': madmen were then regarded simply as
dangerous people on the same level as criminals, debauchees and
beggars. They were therefore excluded from society and 'confined'
along with the other categories of the asocial, often in the same
institutions. There were, of course, charitable people, such as St
Vincent de Paul, who were concerned with improving the plight of
these prisoners, but their philanthropy remained within the framework of the institution; it did not try to break it. Even at the
beginning of the nineteenth century, Maxime du Camp could write:

> The conditions in the Bicêtre asylum at that time were
> unimaginable; it was like a medieval prison in its most hideous
> form: it was a gaol, a poor-house, a penitentiary and a hospital
> all in one. Murderers, bawds, invalids, paupers and half-wits
> were piled together in the most outrageous promiscuity; in a
> word it was a sewer.[1]

Ey tried to discover the ideology underlying this 'alienation' of
the insane. The madman, he wrote, plays the part of a stranger in
our midst: 'he is the man from another world'. Consequently, as
long as the ideology of our society was a religious one, the madman,
because he no longer belonged to society, was considered part of
the supernatural realm. The new ideology that emerged with the
Reformation and the Age of Enlightenment and finally triumphed
with the French Revolution was an ideology of individual freedom.
The madman became the man who had lost his freedom. It thus
becomes clear how the community and the doctors were led into
'alienating' him, banishing him in fact from a society where everything rested on individual freedom and responsibility.[2] The reforms
instituted in France by Pinel, Tuke and Daquin have been described
as a genuine revolution in the care of the mentally ill. It is true that
their chains were removed and their dignity as human beings
restored, but this was no more than a philanthropic gesture.
Meanwhile, the first genuinely scientific conception of insanity was
developing in quite the opposite direction: it aimed to show
that the insane were radically different from other men. Far from
disappearing, the alienating process was reinforced by this new
development. However, the justification given for confining the
insane was changed. It was now deemed necessary, in Esquirol's
words, 'to break all the habits of the lunatic by taking him away

186

from home, separating him from his family, his friends and his servants, surrounding him with strangers and changing his whole way of life'. It is not until the first half of the twentieth century that we witness what Ey calls the 'second psychiatric revolution', characterized by the discovery of the neuroses and of different degrees of severity of the psychoses, and by a shift in interest from the illness to the patient. Psychiatrists then became concerned with 'opening' the asylums and treating the mentally ill, not as people for ever cut off from others, but as an integral part of society.

But have the opinions of the layman always been in step with the evolution of psychiatry? Pélicier attempted to throw light on this question by defining the collective representations of madness prevalent at different times: madness is a festival—as celebrated by Erasmus and Cervantes (the jester, the happy fool, the village idiot, Don Quixote, etc.); madness is a mystery (the trance, the 'sacred disease'); madness is a threat, incurable because of its hereditary nature, a danger to the community and the individual:

> In its three aspects of festival, mystery and threat, madness
> has always been embarrassing to society. This embarrassment
> explains the continual swing of collective attitudes from
> tolerance to condemnation, from incarceration to liberal
> policies. Often in this process the psychiatrist's attitude has
> gone in the opposite direction to that of the collective, his
> austerity denying the festive aspect of madness, his scientific
> approach the mystery and his philanthropy the threat. It is
> obvious, however, that there is a dialectical relationship
> between the ideas of the community and those of the
> psychiatrist.

Although he may be opposed to the ideas of his time, the psychiatrist is very much open to their influence. However, it is the other aspect of the dialectic which seems to us to be more important today: to what extent have the opinions of psychiatrists, aided by the powerful means of propaganda at their disposal, such as radio, television and the Press, changed the opinion of the layman? What conception do ordinary people have today about madness and the people who treat it? This is the more important factor for a structuralist study that wishes to consider the part played by the mentally ill in the social system. Research on this subject comes mainly from the U.S.A.[3] Most of the studies seem to conclude that the scientific approach tends to prevail more and more over the old beliefs, in spite of the fact that the sick person or his relatives still have great difficulty in recognizing serious symptoms or in describing them verbally. It also seems as though the negative attitude of the older generation towards psychiatry is diminishing. However, one should not be over-optimistic. To begin with, the results of investigations vary according to the ethnic *milieu*. They are not the same, for example, for the Anglo-Saxon population of Boston and for the Indians of French Canada: the latter still show the same feelings of anxiety and even of guilt when faced with mental illness as they did in the past; many pathological traits are considered 'normal' and are sometimes even highly valued, such as depression, alcoholism or paranoid schizophrenia. In the second place, the results vary according to sex: women tend to reject organic explanations in favour of environmental ones, while the opposite is true for men; men show panic reactions when faced with mental illness, while women tend to have a charitable attitude towards the insane. Even general practitioners tend to have the same negative attitudes to psychiatric treatment as the lay public: they regard the mentally ill as dangerous people who have entirely lost their mental faculties and are prone to unpredictable behaviour. Some surveys have even shown that the efforts made to spread modern ideas about 'madness' tend to go against the intentions of their promoters: they make people even more anxious, and this anxiety has a harmful effect on mental health.

It appears, therefore, that knowledge about mental illness does not follow a highly organized plan. Attitudes recorded by investigators, even within one community, are extremely varied. Nor is this information crystallized, since individuals tend to change their opinions. There does appear to be a tendency for intellectuals and younger people to be better-informed, but the old conceptions persist and there are often conflicting attitudes within the community. Above all, there is a contrast between the information received, which is more or less positively oriented, and the attitudes of the public, which remain relatively negative. People still look upon the mentally ill with fear and revulsion; they regard them as liars or dangerous people—a different species. Madness, like cancer, is still a shameful disease in the eyes of the public, something to keep hidden.

Doctor and patient. There are some inspiring studies in this field such as Valabrega's *La Relation Thérapeutique*[4] or Récamier's article, 'L'Hystérie et le Théâtre'.[5] However, we cannot make use of them here, as they deal with the relationship between individuals, whereas we, who are dealing with sociology, are deliberately placing ourselves within the structures of society as a whole.

On the other hand, we have efforts, such as Jane Philips's, to construct models of the process of cure according to different civilizations (an attempt which was apparently rather badly received). Her model is expressed in symbolic language by the formula:

$$TS\,[f\,(p+c)] = VSr/s$$

where T denotes technology, f faith, p the applied techniques of physical therapy, c of chemical therapy, V the system of cultural or ethical values, r the totality of roles and s the social structure.[6] Although this sort of approach is more oriented towards the structures and values of society as a whole, it is still not very helpful to us.

The only thing we will retain from this first group of studies is the interrelational definition of illness given by Valabrega: 'Illness is something that happens between the doctor and the patient'. He means by this that illness is not an autonomous entity, but a result of the confrontation of two individuals, the first contributing the mystery of his illness and the second proposing an explanation and fitting the subjective realm into the objectivity of a theoretical system. This very general definition of illness reveals to us that madness does not exist as such, but is a construction growing out of a dialogue. However, the construction transcends the dialogue, since behind the patient is the whole weight of collective representations which he and his friends and relatives have of mental illness, and behind the doctor are the systems he has learnt in books and during his training. The therapeutic dialogue is therefore an exchange between two elements of society rather than two individuals. The substitution, in the psychoanalysis of Lacan, of the realm of language for the realm of things leads us to the same conclusion.[7] The unconscious mind of the patient is no longer regarded as a reservoir of repressed desires, but as part of a discourse which remains hidden, but does leave more or less well-preserved traces, thus giving the analyst a role similar to that of the historian deciphering inscriptions on a monument or translating documents from archives. It is never the patient's symptoms in any case that are analysed, but his words. The use of words, no matter how distorted and subjectivized, implies the introduction of society into the dialogue. From a sociological point of view, psychoanalysis must always be seen as a study of language in a face-to-face situation. In our opinion, by bringing out the linguistic aspect of psychoanalysis, Lacan has illustrated the progress linguistics has brought to the understanding of mental disorder. He has enabled us to see that mental disorder is a communication process, different, perhaps, from other so-called normal processes, but of the same basic nature.

Group therapy complicates the picture somewhat, but the increase in the number of participants only brings out more strongly the importance of communication: the therapeutic group is above all a network of social relations in embryo. The group-therapy situation, at least in some of its forms and according to some authors, brings about the formation of a 'group spirit'; this is particularly noticeable when a patient is transferred from one group to another. Each group has its own particular system of drama-tization and symbolization, its own superego, which is in fact the conscience the group evolves of its own accord, and naturally its own system of censorship and repression.[8] The therapist can, of course, manipulate these communication networks, but if we were to eliminate him we would be left with a genuine 'society of the mentally ill'.

In point of fact, this society is artificial: mentally-ill people do not deliberately come together; they are part and parcel of society and 'communicate' or form networks with normal people. Earlier we mentioned *folie à deux* and group psychosis. The phenomena psychiatrists define in these terms are relatively rare. What more generally occurs is that illness becomes 'ramified' through com-munication networks and affects in one form or another a whole group. This is usually the family group, but it can also be the neighbourhood or occupational group. This phenomenon was well understood by Moreno: his psychodrama treats, either in the form of ego-auxiliaries or directly, not only the patient but also his wife, his children and his wife's friends.[9] We have witnessed a barely perceptible shift from the idea of a deviant individual to the idea of marginal groups evolving within society as a whole or, to be more precise, on the fringe of society. 'People in the immediate surroundings of a catatonic themselves become rigid';[10] faced with a paranoiac, they become aggressive.

We are beginning to distinguish the outlines of a pathological society, but it is, of course, in the mental hospital that its general pattern can be seen most clearly. The policy of locked doors which developed, as we saw in the first part of this chapter, with the change in collective representations of madness consists in separ-ating the patient from society, shutting him up in a closed world, 'isolating' him. The study of the hospital as an institution is probably one of the commonest fields in contemporary sociology. The reasons for this are obvious enough: since the patients are concentrated within a restricted area and separated from the rest of the world, the number of variables is greatly reduced in com-parison with normal society. The patients' activities are greatly limited in scope and nearly always observable; it is therefore possible to examine social interaction without much difficulty—and even to manipulate it. What is more, the toleration in mental hospitals of the direct expression of feelings and attitudes makes it feasible to study these phenomena in their natural state—or at least with fewer disguises.[11] We are not concerned here with knowing whether the hospital, by maintaining the safety of the patient and removing his social responsibilities, is effective, therapeutically speaking, as Devereux and Le Guillant maintain, or whether, on the contrary, it is an instrument of degradation, a systematic cultivation of insanity, or that there is such a thing as a 'sociopathology of the hospital ward', as suggested by Daumezon, Tosquelle, Paumelle and Hermann Simon.[12] It is up to the psychiatrist, on the basis of his experience, to make the necessary value-judgments. The aspect of hospitals which is of interest to the sociologist is the disappearance of ordinary interaction processes. The patient no longer has any familial relations, and even sexual activities are theoretically forbidden; he is deprived of his professional life, and even if he takes part in occupational therapy he is not paid for the work he does. He also enters a new, strongly hierarchical society where mobility is blocked and communication is structured. This led Caudill to suggest a geological analogy: there are two separate strata in the hospital system, the patients on the one hand and the doctors, administrators and nurses on the other. Only formal relations can take place between the two superimposed strata. The only person who can play the role of mediator between them is the nurse, if he is willing and not too overworked. If he does not fulfil this role, the emotional side of the patient's personality becomes disturbed, and this disturbance is manifested either individually (as in the agitation of manic patients, the escape into phantasy of the schizophrenic, who withdraws more and more into his impassive shell) or in a collective way (disturbances of an entire ward). Psychiatrists and sociologists have probably been struck mainly by the negative aspects of hospital life: they have tended to show the role played by the stereotypes governing this society of human debris, e.g. the image of the madman which unconsciously affects behaviour and is often actualized. Or else they have emphasized the physical surroundings: the high walls, the locked doors, the mechanical exercising in the grey, prison-like courtyard. Finally, they have drawn attention to the existence of a sort of public opinion of the mental hospital, where every patient has a reputation to keep up and acts according to what his fellow patients, nurses and doctors will think of him.

Hospital patients could be studied as groups in the same way that anthropologists study small traditional groups. In communities of mental patients one finds processes similar to those studied by Gluckman in South Africa under the name of 'rituals of rebellion'. These are compensatory ceremonies designed to relieve the tensions caused by the rigidity of the social structure. On festive occasions,

191

such as the setting up of the Christmas tree, or during recreative sessions, the gulf is bridged between the two worlds, the doctors and the administrators on the one hand and the patients on the other: the cast line, so to speak, is broken.

Although vertical mobility is impossible, there are still ways, as in ordinary societies, of ascending part of the ladder. For example, a patient whose case is 'interesting' gets special treatment from the staff; psychotherapy is regarded as a promotion because it is so often a 'rich man's treatment'. The same is true for group-therapy, which is a democratic situation where patients are given attention irrespective of ethnic origin, social class, paying or non-paying status. The two anthropological concepts used by Linton, 'role' and 'status', are increasingly being applied in psychiatric research. In France Récamier recognized the value of this change in terminology, which implies the replacement of the vague notion of sociability by that of social status, ambiguous though the status of a patient may be. He writes, for example: 'The mental state and the behaviour of the patient change when his social status changes or is liable to change; they remain fixed when his status itself is fixed.' Courchet, on the other hand, bases himself on Lévi-Strauss's idea of permanent unconscious structures which can be discovered by eliminating 'by a process of filtering . . . the lexicological content of institutions and customs'. He discovered that the dualistic pattern is reflected in the patients' attitudes: the authority figures in the hospital are split into 'friends' and 'enemies', the two halves being complementary—for even the enemy is only an enemy the better to cure one. Finally, it may be possible to say that, just as in traditional societies the dead are linked to the living to form one and the same reality, so in the hospital the phantasies of the patients are an integral part of the reality of the hospital and are involved in all communication networks.

However, social relations still remain asymmetrical, since we are dealing with a stratified society and the patients themselves are more or less seriously ill. Some sort of exchange does take place (money, cigarettes, books, goods smuggled in or stolen from the kitchen), but in face-to-face relations the less ill of the two people involved becomes the protector and guide of the other, rolls his cigarettes, etc. The restricted life of the hospital creates favourable conditions for solidarity on an exchange basis—as in traditional societies with small populations and a limited number of groups. The hospital presents this dualism on many different planes, like a gallery of mirrors: there is a dichotomy between male and female wards, between the area under supervision and the fringe areas where one can more or less escape the attention of the nurses, between the medical regulations (which are the same for all patients, irrespective of the nature of their ailment, of sex, age, marital status or religion) and the regulations of private life, which are marginal to the hospital regulations and consist of ruses, such as smoking cigarettes in the lavatory, love-play in hidden corners when there is an excuse for leaving the ward, etc. The social life of the patient is not determined solely by the organization of the institution, but also by the formation of spontaneous groups (even if the groups are deluded, like Napoleon surrounded by his field-marshals). It must be viewed in terms of the dualism characteristic of all closed communities. The sociology of the hospital leads to the study of structural models.

The Reintegration of the Rehabilitated. Owing to the influence of such men as Bierer, Tosquelles, Sivadon and Lambo, the mental hospital is progressively opening its gates. Stepping-stones are being created between the hospital and the community, such as after-care hostels. The existing environment is exploited to facilitate the readjustment of mental patients (e.g. placement on local farms). The result of this movement is a third type of research concerned with the reintegration of ex-mental patients into occupational and family settings. Social readjustment is largely defined in terms of occupational success: some 'rehabilitated' psychotic patients are even able to gain higher professional qualifications than before they were hospitalized. The reason occupational success is given so much importance is that to a large extent the patient can only take his place in his family if he has a salary to contribute and can show his relatives that he is capable of doing something. However, it is important to differentiate between the conjugal family and the parental family. It is only the former that refuses to take back the patient until he is able to work; the parental family accepts the patient who cannot readjust to an occupation, since his role as the dependent and assisted 'child' is the only one his parents expect.[13]

A recent study in Boston, which dealt with male subjects only, confirms the need to take into consideration both parental and conjugal families when assessing 'social success'. (See Table 27.)

To conclude this review of research, we shall refer to Parsons' classic work on the doctor-patient relationship, which we mentioned at the end of the historical review in Chapter I.[14] Parsons tried to see this relationship in the context of the total social structure and to fit it into a general theory of structural models. His hypothesis is that the patient is a deviant and the doctor an instrument of 'social control'. In other words, the relationship between mental illness and psychiatry is only one particular aspect of the general theory of the relationship between motivation to deviance and mechanisms of control:

193

Table 27 Relationship between combined social and occupational success ratings and type of family[15]

Success rating		Type of family	
Occupational	Social	Parental	Conjugal
High	High	19·0	63·2
High	Low	19·0	26·5
Low	High	8·0	2·9
Low	Low	54·0	7·4
		100·0	100·0

The sick role is, as we have seen, in these terms a mechanism which in the first instance channels deviance so that the two most dangerous potentialities, namely, group formation and successful establishment of the claim to legitimacy are avoided. The sick are tied up, not with other deviants to form a 'sub-culture of the sick', but each with a group of non-sick, his personal circle and, above all, physicians. The sick thus become a statistical status class and are deprived of the possibility of forming a solid collectivity. Furthermore, to be sick is by definition to be in an undesirable state. . . .

He adds that, from this point of view also

In any case such an increase [in mental disorder] need not, as is very commonly asserted, be a direct index of increasing social disorganization. It is quite possible that it constitutes the diversion into the sick role of elements of deviant motivation which might have been expressed in alternative roles. From the point of view of the stability of the social system, the sick role may be less dangerous than some of the alternatives.[16]

We now need to re-examine our issue from this particular angle. But we must point out that the role of the mental patient does not in the slightest eliminate the 'two most dangerous potentialities' that Parsons mentions. First, because the patient's intention is to establish his legitimacy: he believes it is other people who are mad. Secondly, the mental hospital creates the deviant group in order to segregate it from the rest of society. The doctor does, of course, act as an instrument of social control, since he is the person who reveals the patient's subjectivity (as opposed to his legitimacy) and who can open—or partly open—the hospital doors. But even so Parsons's model has to be made somewhat more complex. Moreover, although the alternative ways of expressing deviance are such phenomena as suicide, prostitution or crime, mental illness is probably no less dangerous than these, at any rate to the morale of the community. The proof is that society responds in the same way to all these forms of deviance: by locking up the offender (or, in the case of suicide, by supervision, which is the equivalent of prison without bars).

2 Madness in relation to society

In a previous chapter we asked: What is a case? How can we distinguish between normal and pathological states? We can probably see more clearly now that the reason this question arose was that madness (we deliberately use in this chapter the vague term which psychiatrists would like to exorcise) does not in fact exist as a natural entity, but only as a relationship. The historians rightly transferred madness from the natural to the historical field by defining it in terms of the changing dialogue between the rational and the irrational. Thus we come to the first postulate of structuralism: a person is mad only in relation to a given society; social consensus defines the fluctuating boundary between the rational and the irrational.

In Foucault's terms, 'To write a history of madness is to give a structural picture of a historical totality composed of the concepts, institutions, legal and police practices and scientific concepts which pin down a madness whose primitive state can never actually be recaptured.'

Henri Ey, whose ideas we mentioned previously, clarifies one aspect alone of this structural totality: the field of concepts. He deals particularly with philosophical, political or ethical concepts, such as freedom and responsibility. Institutions and judicial practices are shown to be the consequences of ideologies and not the elements of a structure of which the insane are themselves a part. He thus introduces the causality principle to history and returns us to the issue: Which is the more important, the realm of thought or the infrastructure? Other writers tend to place greater emphasis on the sequence of economic upheavals marking the change from the era of the corporation to the era of the factory, the growth of unemployment and vagrancy, and the formation of a whole marginal urban class that produces tramps, prostitutes, criminals and madmen.

This is the second aspect of those structural totalities which we are now attempting to grasp. The insane cannot be separated from other categories of deviant. Deviance can of course take different forms, depending no doubt on the individual constitution, but also on the social group.[17] However, the various manifestations of deviance, as it has so often been pointed out, show strong deterministic analogies and a tendency to be complementary. (Thus statistical studies show that for a given society or group the suicide curve is often the reverse of the crime curve.) All societies tend, as it were, to secrete and eliminate waste products. Although we are aware of the spurious nature of comparisons between social and biological organisms, it is obvious all the same that the social organism, to be able to function in a harmonious way, has to reject everything its live tissue cannot absorb. Perhaps sociologists ought to take a closer look at the streets of a city in the early morning: the dustbins are being emptied, only to be refilled and re-emptied of everything that each social cell, each family or dwelling unit repeatedly assigns to destruction. They would merely need to take a walk in a town that dates from Roman times to notice the tremendous difference in level between the Roman town and the contemporary town—modern cities are built on the detritus of past generations. A sociology of dustbins has yet to be invented.

As a contemporary science, it would have to be based on the consideration that we live in an industrial society and that our ideology is based on production: deviance is therefore defined in terms of our system of production. Insanity is above all a form of unproductiveness. This is what Sivadon foresaw when he wrote: 'Insanity is the price man has to pay for his noble endeavour always to progress.' But the deepest insight into this question comes, not from a psychiatrist, but from a writer, Béguin. In his preface to an issue of *Esprit* on the 'poverty of psychiatry', he writes: 'The range of behaviour regarded as normal has been narrowed down to that which is compatible with the idea of usefulness and of the good of the community.'

From this viewpoint the opening of the asylums was not so much a philanthropic measure or, as Ey described it, the result of an intense feeling for the dignity of the individual, as a mere desire to fit the deviant into the great machine of society so that he could produce more goods. It is not surprising that the British school of social psychiatry and certain trends in French psychiatry define social success essentially as occupational success. Drug treatment, as lobotomy had done previously, came just at the right moment to facilitate the 'gentle' reintegration of patients into the system of production by eliminating the more aggressive forms of reaction. The reason why tranquillizers or 'chemical strait-jackets' are so widely used is not only, nor even mainly, in spite of what has been said, because of overcrowding in hospitals—which prevents genuine relations from being established between doctor and patient. Neither are they a means of relieving the doctor of his guilt. (With drugs the doctor feels that he has done everything he can. If recovery does not take place, then it is the patient's own fault.) In our opinion, the explanation lies at a deeper level: the whole of society is exerting pressure on the patient; it is only interested in him as a productive element. Whether he is cured or not is irrelevant as long as he can be 'useful'. Drug treatment becomes what the rag-and-bone trade is to the sociology of dustbins: it tries to salvage from the debris anything left of any industrial or commercial value, no matter how limited, so as to put it back into the circuit of production and distribution. The reason we are able to make this statement is that drug treatment is not a recent invention. The *shamans* and priests of sects practising initiation use plants from which present-day remedies are extracted (or plants with similar therapeutic properties) for their ritualistic 'herbal baths', which provoke states of ecstasy. Their aim is to be able thus to 'control' the asocial behaviour of the psychotics so that they become co-operative subjects. 'The good of the community', in the highest sense of the term, becomes the ultimate aim; the disturbed equilibrium of the group must be restored. Psychiatry today is rediscovering these old remedies. In our society, where everyone has to work, it is essential that no manpower should be lost, as it was in the past, through the policy of confinement. 'Usefulness' has replaced 'the good of the community'. Of course, it can be argued that the reintegration of patients into the working community is of philanthropic value; but is philanthropy the motivation behind this policy? The abolition of slavery was also an act of philanthropy much fought for by humanitarians. But in the end slavery was only abolished (let us not forget that it was a voluntary act on the part of the white population and not the result of a Negro revolt) when the development of capitalism showed that slaves were more expensive to keep and less productive than free workers, and when increasing production made it necessary to eliminate that part of the population who, having no salary, could not become consumers.

The very definition we have given of the normal and the pathological is inherent in this technocratic ideology. While the old definition in terms of adjustment is appropriate for a relatively stable industrial society, the new definition in terms of normativeness applies best to our contemporary society. The tremendous pace of technological change, which shifts workers from one sector of production to another completely unrelated sector, requires not adaptation, but adaptability—what the psychologist would call 'plasticity'. The aim of the psychiatrist is to find a niche for the 'rehabilitated' patient, ranging from handicrafts for the mentally defective or epileptic patient to all the other forms of industrial work. It seems, however, that in our world of increasing urbanization, rural exodus and industrialization of agriculture, policy-makers have dropped the custom prevalent only a few years ago of placing ex-patients in 'rural colonies', where they could benefit from contact with Nature and from the company of friendly beasts.

A sociology of insanity needs to articulate insanity with the entire social system. Structuralism has the merit of preserving integrally the conclusions of our previous chapters by transforming the causal links, so often the object of debate between geneticists, biologists and sociologists, into correlative links. But these correlations have a specific orientation, since both mental disturbance and normal states are a function of a collective order which, as Lévi-Strauss pointed out, is affected even by the exception. Those who, for one reason or another, find themselves outside the system are 'expected and even forced' to work out compromises or imaginary syntheses between the various contradictory elements of the system. Inevitably 'History introduces allogenic elements into these systems; it produces shifts from one type of society to another and discrepancies between the rhythms of evolution of each particular system'. It is therefore not surprising that the insane, along with criminals, have been classified by 'social pathologists' as 'marginal'.

Let us return to our own society, which we have defined as a society of *Homines fabri*. Max Weber's excellent analysis showed that its main characteristic relative to earlier societies is the growing importance played by rationalization. Mannheim, in spite of his concern with preserving human values, had to admit that the scientific exploitation of Nature tends towards totalitarian planning. We are being engulfed little by little in a world of technology, machines, 'functional' housing and organized leisure. But there still remain within our wider social system whole sections of society condemned to death which could be called 'sacred societies'. In his preface to the special issue of *Esprit* mentioned above, Béguin puts this very well: from Nietzsche to Antonin Artaud, the madman has always pointed an accusing finger at society. When rationalism began to hold sway at the time of the Renaissance, Erasmus could be content with writing a treatise in *Praise of Folly*. But today we need to go further: it is necessary for us to become madmen to discredit a society that has itself gone mad. Nietzsche tried to break the wheel of technical existence—that is, the conditioning of means to ends—first by exhorting us to turn our scale of values upside-down and then by living this reversal himself through the model of madness. For Gérard de Nerval and Antonin Artaud insanity is a protest against the doctors who 'make sure the realm of poetry does not spread to the streets'. Madness has a 'sociological' significance in that it brings to light the clash within society as a whole between two systems belonging to different eras: *techne* and *poiesis*.

Bachelard, who is a philosopher, not a sociologist, tries to save both systems, rationalism and poetry, by assigning to each a different sphere of our life or our personality. The sociologist, on the other hand, is forced into the realization that such phenomena as relaxation therapy, yoga or mass culture change *poiesis* into *techne*, for if poetry is to be changed into a counter-technique, it will necessarily become technicized. There is no solution other than the absurd. It is not without justification that modern painting has been compared to the work of madmen and the language of psychotics to *lettrisme*. Whereas the comparison is not valid aesthetically speaking, it makes sense in sociological terms. We find the same resistant nuclei of the sacred realm reverting to its 'primitive' state, the same peripheral zone in relation to the dominant system of our society, the same archaic systems suddenly exasperated by the insidious gnawing of the central zone of which they are the objects and the victims. The madman is conscious of the impossibility of linking two opposite systems belonging to two different eras. *Poiesis* either becomes *techne* by a process of contamination, or else it stands as a condemnation—a useless one, since all communication is severed and the words of the insane fall on deaf ears. We cannot help admiring this desperate solution. It is the only real solution, since all the other nuclei, such as surrealism, dadaism, abstract art, concrete poetry, are only hypocritical solutions, harmless (and lucrative) ways of playing at madness, indulged in by *bourgeois* and candidates for the *bourgeoisie*, and therefore part of the system of commercial production. Of course, the duality of *poiesis* and *techne* does not exhaust the question of the marginality of the insane. We mentioned it as an example. The technical world excludes other values, such as affectivity,[18] irrationality, the concept of the individual's 'subjectivity'. Madness can be regarded as a resistant enclave of affectivity, myth and pure subjectivity within the dominant system. We could have concentrated on other sociological dimensions, such as the duality of 'community' and 'society'. The madman is never isolated, since he exists in dialectical relationship with his relatives and neighbours. He affects them as well as

199

being affected by them: he uses emotional blackmail on others, manipulates his parents and friends and encloses them within his own world. He is both disturbed and disturbing to them. The remains of the community system in our urban industrialized society take on the aspect of a minority group in a multiracial society; that is to say, it bears the 'mark of oppression' conferred by the rest of society. This provokes the scotomization and petrification of the community elements: they become fossilized. However, it is not necessary to dwell on this subject further, as our first example is enough to show what is meant by compromises and abortive syntheses between systems. The isolation which for some psychiatrists characterizes the world of the mentally ill is merely the translation, in morphological terms, of the marginality of values that have been rejected or repressed by the rest of society. It represents an effort to find a 'niche' in the structure of social space, where these values can hide and vegetate, and where they can defend themselves by secreting a shell which finally reduces to its bare existential minimum what it was intended to preserve.

The concept of schizophrenia has sometimes been attacked by psychiatrists, who maintain that it is of little nosological value. This is not for us, but for the psychiatrists, to debate; however, we can state with confidence that schizophrenia constitutes a genuine sociological category. It is an excellent definition of people living in niches; it also describes the situation we mentioned earlier where the individual secretes a rigid shell to protect his value-systems in a dormant and protoplasmic form against the attacks of a hostile social system.

Little by little, as we have been situating various systems in relation to each other, we have emerged from the problem of the relative position of these systems into the domain of values and significations which will be the central point of our next chapter. We shall therefore return shortly to the points we have just touched on to view them in terms of the communication between central and marginal areas. Nevertheless, the allusion we made to values was necessary to explain why the central system leads to the creation of dispersed peripheral nuclei. The setting up of an ideal by society necessarily creates residues that are non-integrated and finally even rejected because of the danger they represent to the accepted values of the masses. From the social psychiatric point of view, insanity is a disturbance of the personality or of behaviour whose origin must be discovered (by weighing up the various factors that have a part in this genesis). From the point of view of structuralist sociology, insanity is an 'institution' operating within an institutional framework. The role of parents or marriage partners, judges or doctors, guided either by custom or by the written law, is to decide (with the aid of criteria differing according to social class, family income and the public interest) in which sociological category the sick person is to be placed. They thus provide a 'niche', ranging from a bed in a large mental hospital to a position in a small workshop or on an isolated farm. Even by opening the doors of the asylum they are only substituting niches closer to the central nucleus for more peripheral niches. The relapsed patient is the exact equivalent of the criminal recidivist, just as after-care establishments correspond to probation for delinquents; they represent criteria which permit more accurate allocation within a given social system. Since our present system is a rationally planned one, we could call these phenomena a 'planned tolerance of insanity'.

Clearly, one is insane only in relation to a particular society. One of the most interesting conclusions of structuralism is to show that dualities can only be understood with reference to a third term, which may be latent, but which analysis must discover. For example, a structural study of race relations must not only take into account, as previously, Ego and his prejudices and Alter, his victim, the Negro, but also the public; in other words, what the rest of society expects of Ego. In relation to shamanism, Lévi-Strauss points out that the patient treated by the *shaman* is possibly the least important aspect of the system; the crucial relationship is that between the *shaman* and the community. The therapeutic process always extends beyond the duality of doctor and patient and introduces, as a mediator between the two, the social group. No true recovery can take place without the 'consensus' of the community. We have seen in the present chapter how the same is true of contemporary society: we always need to introduce a third term to be able to understand psychopathological systems. The psychiatrist is dependent on society: it provides him with a definition of mental illness, erects an ideal which guides his treatment of it, and decides what goals he shall pursue. The link uniting him with his patient is relatively unimportant. What Lévi-Strauss said of shamanism can also be said of present-day psychiatry: the collective consensus defines insanity and decides when it is cured; in the system of madness the 'madman' is the least important element.

We could give many illustrations of this principle, but one is particularly worthy of mention; it is the most significant because it touches on two different 'publics'. It has been observed that psychiatrists who treat Africans in Europe use a sort of 'white magic' against the black magic of mental illness. In this counter-witchcraft the psychiatrist has the support of the entire white European public: his white magic corresponds to so-called scientific, rational medicine, which society unanimously accepts. And yet, while it succeeds for white patients, it most often fails in the case of Africans. (Even drug treatment fails, although in theory it should be effective, since Europeans and Africans are physiologically identical: neurotic or psychotic symptoms reappear immediately.) But the patient dismissed as 'incurable' needs only to be repatriated to Africa and to receive treatment from a witch-doctor for his disturbances to disappear for good. The difference is that he has now found his own 'public'; he falls back into line with the collective consensus of his fellow Africans. He could not be cured in Europe, since his native culture prevented him from being integrated into a consensus based on values different from his own ethnic values. This shows clearly how the third term which remains concealed, the public, is more important than the two visible links in the chain, the patient and the doctor.

The function of the sociology of mental disorder, as we tried to show in the second part of this chapter, consists in throwing light on this third term; it links the 'insane' and those who treat them with the wider field that defines both the criteria of madness and the criteria of recovery.

XI   The world of 'madness'

1   Towards a structuralist sociology

In the previous chapter we saw that the mentally ill cannot be located within society as a whole unless we recognize the structures of deviant systems in relation to the structure of the main system. Up to now we have only taken what was in a sense a negative view of these deviant systems in opposition to the main system. We now need to penetrate, as sociologists, into the 'world of madness'. Here again we have many excellent studies at our disposal, the results of which must be reviewed before we can see how they fit together or provide the material for a sociological synthesis.

Although it has become fashionable, at least in French psychiatric circles, to criticize Charles Blondel's theories in *La Conscience Morbide*, we have to admit that he was the first to evolve a sociology of mental disorder that was not aetiologically-oriented, but structuralist. His point of view was similar to the one we are now adopting: mental illness is a disturbance, not of the individual, but of communication. However, it was not until the Americans rediscovered this idea that it definitively took root.[1] Sociological theory has, of course, changed since Blondel's time. There is no need to trace here the progression from the study of collective representations (or, in the case of madness, individual representations which tend to be dependent on collective ones) to the study of their origin: man defined by his symbolic activity. The important fact is that any theory of symbolism necessarily includes a pathology. This pathology has two different aspects. The first will not concern us here (signs operate to create, not only co-operative, but also competitive behaviour; symbols exaggerate conflict and justify forms of slavery). The second aspect will be the focal point of this chapter: symbols have different meanings for normal and mentally-ill people; for the former they facilitate communication and for the latter they obstruct it.[2]

The most penetrating studies in this field have been made on schizophrenia. Bleuler defined schizophrenia as a loss of vital contact with reality—that is, autism. But the isolation is not absolute: in some cases the outside world is effectively neutralized, while in others, on the contrary, it is experienced as hostile. Récamier went so far to say—and we believe he is right—that although the schizophrenic may seem at first sight to be cut off from the social community, there is probably no one more vulnerable to external human influences. 'The indifference of the schizophrenic is only real because the environment responds by indifference to the false protective indifference of the sick person struggling with the fundamental experience of his psychosis.' The schizophrenic's fear of the world is proportional to the attraction it holds for him; he fuses with it and loses in the process his own individuality to the extent that if 'the other withdraws, he is left with nothing'.[3]

From another point of view, Minkowski showed that, as well as the impoverished autism characterized by stereotyped and rigid inner phantasies, there is a florid type of autism comparable to the world of dreams, characterized by a profusion of phantasies, like a bouquet of strange flowers. The latter form of autism is the one described by Kretschmer when he compares the schizophrenic to a house with bare whitewashed walls and hermetically drawn curtains, hence having no exchange with the outside world, within which sumptuous feasts take place.[4] However, whenever we are able to gain access to the 'feast', the striking thing about the world of the psychotic is its rationalism and geometrism. The sick person cannot assimilate any movement or life, and tends to build his inner world along spatial lines, following rules which we would recognize as belonging specifically to logic and mathematics.[5] American psychiatrists have tended to emphasize both this break with the social world (which they regard not so much as a withdrawal as a failure to play the appropriate roles or as an impairment of the functioning of the ego) and the purely individual and therefore incommunicable symbols which characterize the delusions of the schizophrenic.[6] Cameron in particular draws attention to the creation of an asocial idiom (metonymy) and an arbitrary syntax (asyndesis). However, in his withdrawal from the outside community, the schizophrenic is able (in the case of paranoid behaviour) to recreate the community by attributing to others his own feelings about himself, by organizing people into imaginary behaviour. He transforms the real community into a functional 'pseudo-community' of detractors and persecutors.[7] The pseudo-community of the neurotic, on the other hand, is more likely to be composed of

'Prince Charming' characters, lovelorn maidens and regal or divine father-figures.[8]

However, all that these increasingly fashionable structural analyses are attempting to do is to structure the content of delusional images or apparently absurd modes of behaviour. We must go deeper than this. Earlier we quoted Lévi-Strauss as saying that individual delusions obey the same formal rules as collective myths. This is the second contribution of contemporary science to our sociology of mental disorder: the structuralist approach, which leads us from content to form. Myths can, of course, be explained historically with reference to social realities, rituals and particular situational factors. In the same way, the delusions of a psychotic can always be traced back to the history of an individual. Nevertheless, in both cases these phenomena of the imagination represent autonomous realities constructed according to their own particular rules and principles, which structural analysis must try to discover. Two comments seem worth mentioning, however, as they impose limitations on Lévi-Strauss's statement. The first is from Sebag,[9] who describes pathological symbolism in the individual as

> a perpetual over-turning of syntax and vocabulary. The code
> in which these messages are communicated is subject to sudden
> and total changes, since the conditions of transmission are
> such that the code can only be used by a sole transmitter.
> Moreover, the plasticity of the message to be communicated
> is so pronounced that the syntax used can be of practically
> any order. . . . Individual symbolism reproduces in a microcosm
> all the variants of collective symbolism, but at the same time
> it eliminates part of their specificity. . . . The syntaxes
> intertwine and partly dissolve, the communicated message
> being of such a nature that it can bend itself to any formal
> organization.

This is not to say that formal organization disappears, but while myths retain a certain structural stability which makes their comparison possible, the delusions of the mentally ill juggle with so many different meta-languages that comparison between them is more difficult, if not impossible, given our present state of knowledge.

Our second comment takes us much deeper. A number of psychiatrists, such as Resnik in Argentina and Bobon and Roumeguère in France,[10] have illustrated how words, either written or spoken, are transformed by the mentally ill from symbols into 'objects'. The schizophrenic does not express himself in symbols, but rather it is the psychiatrist who creates symbols from the word-objects. The patient uses these words like toys to dramatize a situation exactly as children do when they play with words. Or else he regards them as dangerous things: he blocks his ear with his finger because listening is incorporating a social food which is sucked in through the ear—or as aggression by magical forces against which he must defend himself. But this sort of observation only really shifts the problem to another level; it does not solve it. If language becomes crystallized into object form, then the 'original signification has to be found elsewhere, beyond the discourse'—for example, in silence. Silence is also a language, and the psychiatrist must learn to read the words that lie behind its various forms. We are dealing with a new meta-language which operates in the form of subtle messages from the body (babies, for example, send out all sorts of information which their mothers are perfectly able to decipher). In all probability, this meta-language also follows structural principles. The schizophrenic, who is afraid of translating his thoughts into words as the words are welded on to his being like live bits of flesh, speaks in spite of himself through his muscular movements and, when he is not moving, through his immobility and silence. But what type of analysis can reveal the formal laws governing these meta-languages? The science of structures still has a long way to go.

The third important contribution of modern science to the development of a sociology of mental disorder is in the field of history and anthropology. History reveals that delusions are not merely the activity of sick people, but collective constructions in which society plays at least as great a part as the sick person himself. For instance, the witch-hunts of the Middle Ages were the product of a constant dialogue between the inquisitors and the alleged witches. Similarly, Charcot's *grande hystérie* at the end of the nineteenth century was more a construction of the medical men than of the hysterics themselves: as soon as the doctors ceased to believe in it, the symptoms elaborated in the course of the dialogue became less frequent or vanished altogether. Hysteria had become a sort of pithiatism. In the same way, anthropology shows that each society has its own 'correct way of going mad' and that this model is furnished by the myths or customs of the people.[11] Devereux emphasized the preconceptions about madness that society evolves and imposes from without, as it were, on the sick person. In other words, madness is a 'social fact' in the Durkheimian sense. The sick person, to be recognized as sick, has to make his behaviour conform to the behaviour traditionally expected of the madman. Psychotics tend to develop the symptomatology that will enable the psychiatrist to classify their disturbances according to socially defined criteria.[12] A Chipewa Indian tends to develop a *windigo* syndrome, a Malayan a *lattah* psychosis. Fundamentally speaking, all madness is a form of *folie à deux* involving the psychiatrist and the patient, in which the psychiatrist represents the public (the collective conceptions of madness) and the patient endeavours to help him make his diagnosis by taking the opposite course to the behaviour of normal people by making his disturbances into a ritual of rebellion.[13] Devereux has given many examples of the traditional models enabling sick people to define themselves as mad, taken from the Bible, Homer (the *Odyssey*, Books 4 and 13) and from his own observation of the Mohave Indians. Nearly every mythology in the world has its mad gods on whom human beings model their aberrant behaviour so as to notify whoever it may concern, the *shaman* or the doctor, the family or the law-court, of their marginal position in society.

This brings us back along a different road to the conclusion of the previous chapter: the dynamics of mental disorder operate within a system where both the deviant and society are in collaboration. In fact, from this point of view we could demonstrate that it is not only the appearance of the illness which is part of the system, but also its disappearance. Recovery is 'recognized' with the aid of criteria which can change from culture to culture (as we mentioned earlier, active participation in the economic system tends to be an increasingly important criterion in our society).[14]

These three perspectives are apparently contradictory. The first emphasizes the break in communication and the opposition between the public realm of normal people and the private realm of the mentally ill: it expresses the judgment of the psychiatrist and corresponds to the scientific definition of mental disorder. The second, on the other hand, suggests that the private realm obeys the same formal laws as the public realm; therefore it expresses the reaction of the anthropologist to the psychiatrist. Unfortunately, we cannot refer to a structuralist analysis of individual myths similar to the analyses made of collective myths; but this, as we suggested, would tend to be a much more difficult task, since it would have to juggle with so many different meta-languages as well as with communication beyond speech. For this reason the second approach will remain more of a project for further research than a contribution to the sociology of mental disorder. The third approach is akin to the second, since it refuses to separate the world of insanity from the world of normal people. The break in communication is real only in appearance. Even in the most serious cases of schizophrenia it is possible to effect a cure if one can transform the object-word into a sign-word or, in Lacan's words, 'the imaginary' into discourse.[15] If 'the imaginary' *can* be transformed into discourse, this is because the world of insanity is an integral part of the greater realm of collective representations—in other words, private symbolism is at some point connected to the network of public

207

symbolism. In reality, the term 'private' applies less to the symbolism itself than to its uses by the sick person. Thus the third approach is related to the second. However, it is more functional. Better still, whereas the second approach leads us to anthropology, the third really places us within the field we have chosen, sociology —that is, not the analytical study of the imaginary, but the study of the dialogue between society and the insane. We shall therefore confine ourselves in the present chapter to this last perspective.

2 Functionalism

We hope the reader will allow us to introduce a digression on functionalism. Far from taking us away from our subject, it will bring us more deeply into it. Psychiatrists have shown the various functions of mental disorder. When existence becomes too complicated and presents too many formidable problems, the individual tends to descend to a lower level of activity: he economizes his gestures or his speech and shrinks his experience to fit his deficiency of psychic resources. When considered from this particular viewpoint, neurosis and psychosis are solutions of some usefulness. But in this case functionalism is a purely pychological approach and cannot be of interest to us. However, there is another type of functionalism, developed by Freud and his followers, which replaces the sick person within the framework of social relations. Pathological behaviour is seen as a sort of blackmail, a means of intimidation, a manipulation of the environment. The neurotic is always threatening to have a breakdown if his friends and relatives try to oppose his wishes. 'There is none so clever as a madman,' as the popular French saying goes. For example, psychoanalysis was able to discover that a particular patient's obsessional rituals were in fact a desire to prevent her father from remarrying by forcing him to keep a constant watch on her behaviour; that the bedtime rituals of a young virgin and the fear that overtook her at the moment of falling asleep represented a wish to prevent her parents from having sexual relations: 'she had simulated fear or used a real fear to ensure that the door separating her parents' room from her own was left open during the night'.[16]

However, morbid symptoms can only affect other people if they can be transformed into messages. The madman or the neurotic communicate with others by means of an apparently paradoxical language. The following text, written by a patient, Nicole, is particularly striking:

> I am now in the world of the lucid. But what I have to say
> cannot be communicated, or only inadequately, with the

vocabulary and syntax of the lucid. . . . So when the lucid and
coherent language disintegrates, when the most desperate,
frenzied movements and the most tragically human pantomime
are defeated by the strait-jacket or by drugs, how can one
entreat, curse or blaspheme?

In the last resort, there is the anus.

Incontinence is not only imbecility and loss of cortical
control; incontinence is a form of plastic expression. It is
plastic expression in its crude and formless form, spurting
forth from the body and the instincts which have become
unburdened and liberated.[17]

The soiling of the body with excreta is an appeal (how else to
entreat?) or a condemnation (how else to blaspheme?). It is not a
return to Nature, but the expression of a particular culture—in
other words, a dialogue with others. This dialogue may take the
form of a condemnation or an act of rebellion of the madman
against an alienating society. It can also be the expression of a
desire to gain a reputation within a marginal group of being the
'perfect madman', the madman who dares to go to the very limits of
absurdity. But in each case madness is not isolation; it is a form of
being-in-the-world. Generally, in fact, it is the simplest solutions
that are resorted to in morbid behaviour, i.e. the reversal of normal
behaviour: screaming, tearing of clothes, incoherent speech, absolute
mutism, total immobility, etc.—in short, a response to all external
stimuli by the opposite of what is expected of the sane person,
thereby signalling one's madness to others. On the other hand,
every culture has its image—or images—of the madman, the half-
wit, the epileptic, the neurotic, the depressive; hence these stereotyped behaviours. Nothing could be more commonplace, more
conformist, more imprisoned in their rigid framework than these
morbid forms of behaviour. It is as though society were winning
more surely just where by definition it should no longer have any
effect. But the stereotype of both delusions and behaviour enables
the patient's friends and relatives to 'classify' him and provokes in
the environment the appropriate responses, such as calling for the
psychiatrist or the police, giving the patient a 'change of air' or
locking him up in the security of the asylum. The language of the
insane may well be a foreign language; it is nevertheless well
understood by normal people. We learn it in the numerous jokes
about lunatics, which are part of our popular culture. Both sides of
the dialogue depart from it as little as possible. The psychiatrist's
concern for a particularly 'interesting' patient may, of course,
stimulate the patient to complicate and embellish his psychosis, to
steer it away from the primitive stereotypy in order to satisfy the

doctor's interest, which flatters his vanity. An analysis of what we described as the patient-doctor *folie à deux* shows that the schizophrenic is always careful not to lose contact. Although he may elaborate on it, basically he accepts the 'spare' personality which has been given him (or which he has conferred on himself, but which others accept). The slightest movement in his surroundings is experienced intensely and responded to according to the logical rules of his psychosis, so that the dialogue can be established.

We have attempted to replace the mentally-ill within the world of language and within society, which is in a sense a continuous exchange of information. These few remarks do not however exhaust the subject. Every society has its spatial and temporal frameworks. Mental disorder is articulated (by a more or less unconscious process, but then all social control operates unconsciously) with these frameworks which are provided, as they are for normal people, from without. The traditional term of 'lunatic', meaning a person whose attacks of mental disturbance come and go with the phases of the moon, was indicative of a rather curious aspect of madness: its periodicity. But the explanation was sought —as it still is among country people—in a meteorological phenomenon and not in social influences. However, even this meteorology is in a sense social, since it rests on the lunar myth and in particular on the idea that the moon (Hecate, the moon-goddess) is linked with all things dangerous to the human race, such as tidal waves, menstrual blood and demonic attacks. It marks the moments in life when disorder creeps into the world, when the female dirties and poisons the male and the madman enters the mysterious realm of the unknown. One may well wonder in this case whether the moon does not act as a mythical moon rather than as a real moon, the latter being merely the stimulus that awakens the old magical images.

There are other periodicities of an even more surprising nature in the incidence of psychosomatic disorders. It is generally preferred to regard them as strange coincidences rather than causal relationships. Inman writes:

> Illnesses beginning at Christmas, like those beginning—or becoming worse—at Easter, are always exciting events to speculate upon. Some day the Church and the medical profession will awake to a realization of the immense amount of clinical material furnished by these two Church festivals, the one dealing with virgin birth and the other with equally amazing phenomena, death and resurrection.

Elsewhere he reports a number of observations of disturbances linked to the celebration of religious festivals—in particular, people who die on Good Friday (which is a Christian form of thanatomia and could well constitute, if it were studied in greater detail, a chapter to add to Mauss's famous essay[18]). In other patients, Good Friday, the day the Son died to appease his angry Father, awakens guilt feelings, with attacks of somatic disturbance which can only really be explained in psychic terms by a desire for self-punishment. Inman concludes:

> I am frequently asked if periodicity affects only certain types of people. The subject is vast and needs prolonged scientific study, especially of a statistical kind. I have to content myself with impressions derived from odd experiences in the last thirty years. Time is a basic structure of life, and, no matter what his mental make-up, man cannot avoid its influence. . . . It would seem as if periodicity was as omnipresent as the Oedipus complex with which it is so commonly associated. Like the complex, however, it may press more heavily upon some individuals than upon others.[19]

According to Inman, those most liable to be affected are obsessionals, hysterics, the morbidly anxious and the manic-depressive.

Thus the Church provides mythical models operating on the individual and imposing a rhythm on his psychic life which even has somatic repercussions. The same remarks could be made about the spatial framework which governs mental disorder just as inevitably as the temporal framework. Naturally, the structuring of space does not happen in the same way with the schizophrenic as with the normal person. The schizophrenic prefers to use the contact receptors (touch, taste) and the proximity receptors (smell) rather than the distance receptors (sight, hearing).[20] But this is in order to restructure space according to a new design related to ideas of symmetry, repetition and absolute homogeneity. A whole system of schizophrenic logic exists which is only absurd because we are not ourselves logical beings. It could easily be shown that the delusional constructions of the schizophrenic obey the same fundamental laws as our mathematical constructions (symmetrical or homothetical figures, figures reversed on their axes, etc.). This is where we can see the appropriateness of Minkowski's use of the term 'geometrism'. It may also be possible to show, as some psychiatrists have done, that the magical figures which are elements of this morbid space resemble certain archetypes of primitive religions. Thus 'Antoine' walks with his palms turned backwards, forming a 'screen', or turned towards his body; his fingers are spread out 'to drain off *la substance*'; he walks in a spiral, like a Dogon peasant ploughing his field, 'to fight against *les élémentaires*' or as a cathartic exercise in imitation of the movement of the cosmos.[21] But these are merely justifications after the act, rationalizations of movements imposed by a particular structuring of space which can be created as much by the real environment as by the mental activity of the patient. In the hospital, with its enclosed courtyard, high walls and locked doors, the patient has no alternative but to walk in a spiral or a circle, to repeat the same route endlessly. His circular perambulations within the rigid rectangle of the asylum can thus quite easily evoke the magic circle of defence (of the town, the individual or the country) which Saintyves observed in his study of Jewish folklore and religion. Space is always structured in relation to a central point: it is therefore not surprising that certain delusions contain ideas analogous to those Mircea Eliade observed in the primitive mentality—the existence of a centre of the world at the point of intersection of the different levels of the cosmos, a 'navel of the universe', a heart of reality and sacredness, situated somewhere in the hospital or in the patient's body. Eliade put this very clearly when he emphasized 'the need man constantly experiences to actualize the archetype right down to the most vile and impure levels'. Here again, however, the mythical images are only the ideologies that sick people have built up from ideas imposed from without. This is obvious in psychotic and neurotic immigrants and displaced persons. Their entire activity (which usually does not show this type of *a posteriori* rationalization) consists in recreating a 'centre' in their new environment—in other words, in reconstructing, in a new space unstructured in their eyes and consequently threatening, the old space, which is reassuring because it is centred (around the house, the enclosed room, the image of the mother's breast).[22]

The 'madman' is often puzzling to ordinary people. Nevertheless, he inhabits the same mental universe as normal man. He fits into the same structural frameworks and sends out to others, to define himself in relation to them, precisely those messages that others expect of the 'madman'. However, the mental universe which is shared by both mad and sane changes with the times. We now need to follow the patterns of this change to see if they are the same for the mentally ill as for normal people.

3 The mental universe of the mad and the sane

One of the patterns emphasized by such anthropologists as Redfield or such sociologists as Bechler is the evolution from the sacred to the profane, the process of 'secularization'. It is commonly known that delusions of a mystical nature, such as lycanthropy or identification with Christ or the Virgin Mary, are becoming more and more rare, giving way to delusions of a scientific nature (electrical discharges, internal radio sets, electronic messages transmitted by the organs, etc.). The Messiahs that used to clutter up our asylums are being replaced by Utopians, fanatical rationalists, builders of systems for eternal peace and, soon perhaps, planners of the world economy.

In Brazil, on the other hand, the author found an important proportion of religious delusions. taking on different hues according to the origin of the patients. Folk Catholicism is the predominant influence among country people, spiritualism among the poor whites in the city, and African religion more or less linked with *candomblé* among the Negroes. Among West Indians in Paris we find a transitional state between the old and the new models, a curious syncretism between electricity and the medieval witchcraft of spell-casters. Behind all these phenomena there may be the same deep-seated coenesthetic disturbance—to use Blondel's term—but expressed in different vocabularies borrowed from the vocabulary of normal people and ensuring that communication is not broken between the marginal and the central zones.

As we said before, all this is common knowledge. However, it can provide us with a point of departure for a deeper analysis of the problem. Secularization is not exactly the same thing as profanation; it detaches certain emotions from sacred objects and confers them on other objects without changing the nature of the emotions. The cult of the dead is continued in the homage paid to the Unknown Soldier; the Tree of Liberty has replaced the maypole and the Hero of the Revolution is canonized in a very similar way to Catholic saints. One would expect a similar phenomenon to occur in the process of secularization of insanity. As Nietsche pointed out, at one time it was possible to take refuge in a convent, but now the only refuge left is madness. The asylum becomes a secularized convent where new liturgies are celebrated by a world which first drove out the great god Pan and is now proceeding to kill the Christian God. To a great extent madness is a sacred illness. This is not because it lowers the mental level of the subject by attacking the more recent levels of thought (according to the famous principle of regression, which may not be quite so valid as it was thought), thus exposing the images of primitive magic or totemism and arousing the archetypes lying dormant like rejected divinities in their purple robes. It is because the secularization of madness, parallel to the secularization of our social behaviour, detaches religious emotion from the 'sacred' and orients it towards the 'profane'. This is not a process of destruction, but of substitution— both in the pathological realm and in our so-called normal society. The only difference is that in normal society the substitution occurs in the outside world, whereas among the mentally ill it takes place in the obscure depths of the personality.

When we compare a primitive community with a modern one, the most striking thing is that in the primitive community the links between the living, the dead and the gods are real. The ancestors haunt the village, communicate with their descendants in dreams or in the shape of masked dancers and join in the rituals of the living. The gods also come down from heaven, ride on the backs of their faithful, speak through their mouths, or create in order to converse with mortals a particular language in the form of animal footprints in the sand, open or closed sea-shells, signs and omens. In our civilization the roads linking the natural with the supernatural have gradually become closed to circulation. At least in the past, on particular days of the year, such as All Saints' Day, the Carnival or Palm Sunday, the army of ghosts and spirits would descend to mingle with ordinary people. Secularization has meant the severing of these very last links. But the dead and the gods are taking their revenge: they have discovered other ways of insinuating themselves into a world that rejects them; they have changed their masks so that no one can recognize them and chase them away. They are making their return in the shape of imagos.[23] But while the dead and the gods were not dangerous, since their coming was under the control of the collective and was governed by strict traditional rules, the new clandestine return of the imagos through the night of the unconscious and no longer in the broad daylight of public festivities is infinitely more dangerous to mental health.

If our previous comments are valid, the secularization of pathological phenomena means that we have exchanged the 'sacred disease' for the wrath of imagos.

> The instinctual representative develops with less interference and more profusely if it is withdrawn by repression from conscious influence. It proliferates in the dark, as it were, and takes on extreme forms of expression, which when they are translated and presented to the neurotic are not only bound to seem alien to him, but frighten him by giving him the picture of an extraordinary and dangerous strength of instinct.[24]

However, in this passage Freud remains within the solitude of the individual libido. The imago appears when imaginative activity substitutes a dream-character for a real character with whom we have a give-and-take relationship. Melanie Klein, who made an excellent study of the imago in children, defines it as a system of representations highly charged with affectivity (either extremely good or extremely bad characters), ranging from the anonymous aggressive images of the very first years of life to the more concrete images of parents and their substitutes typical of the genital phase. In particular she brings to light the imago of the 'devouring being': the one-year-old child is afraid of being devoured and destroyed; he wishes himself to destroy the love-object by biting, devouring and cutting. This imago is the secularized version of the female ogre or cannibalistic monster.[25]

Others have analysed more complicated imagos—for example, the sexual imago of an androgynous being uniting masculine attributes, such as gauntlets, with the silhouette of a mother-figure, the result both of the introjection of the threat of castration by the father and the symbolic projection of virility on to the female partner: the unreal sexual figure is built up of the visual elements of a normative identification with the father, but is destructured.[26] Or, again, the imago of the 'knight saving the maiden from the dragon', which replaces the model of the man-woman relationship prescribed by society by an imaginary model and a 'make-believe' role of liberator, arbiter or righter of wrongs.[27] We are reminded of the words of the poet who had the courage to plunge into the abyss:

> Everything can happen in madness, since all perspective is lost. An idea can only follow one route.[28]

The important thing for us to note is that these imagos, although private creations, enter into the socialized life of the insane exactly as the ancestors and the gods in primitive societies kept up a real and continuous relationship with the living and were an integral part of the village community in the same way as men, women, children and cattle. Modern imagos are the secularized form of the masked priests. In the same way that the anthropologist is able to describe or analyse the avenues of communication between the natural and the supernatural in primitive communities, the psychiatrist can describe the interplay between the imago and the sick person. Thus the restrictions and prohibitions of society can be experienced by the patient as castration; if so, he defends himself against society by a more or less conscious imago of fragmentation (Lebovici and Diatkine). The antidote in this case is to provoke the appearance of an *alter ego* in the group-therapy situation—a secularized version, this time, of the mythical figure of the twin.[29]

Secularization can also occur by another process, in appearance even more anti-religious: the somatization of psychic disturbance. We are dealing here with a projection, not on to imaginary beings, but on to parts of the body, especially the endocrine system (the physiological substratum of the cathexis of the ego by drives and affects) and the digestive system (the earliest locus of sexual drives).[30]

215

The growing importance of psychoses centred on the organs and psychosomatic illnesses in the clinical picture of modern medical science indicates that we are witnessing a metamorphosis of symptoms. The self turns away more and more from the outside world to recapture it in the net of the imaginary, and regresses to the soma which becomes the locus of disturbance. Opler emphasized this somatization in contemporary society as opposed to primitive societies in *Culture, Personality and Human Values*; however, in the same work he points out that somatic symptoms and conversion hysteria are prevalent in primitive cultures, whereas in the Western world psychic disorders are manifested more often in mental disorganization. How can we reconcile these apparently contradictory statements? This is where sociology makes its contribution to psychiatry, by showing how the same disturbance can have different meanings. In non-literate societies there is, in a sense, an excess of the sacred—in other words, tendencies that would be morbid in our society can be objectified and crystallized in external manifestations, in particular in ritual (for example, the development of magic limits the incidence of obsessional neurosis). Under these conditions anything that cannot be objectified tends to become displaced on to the organs of the body. In Western society, on the other hand, as the scientific knowledge of the public develops due to the press, the audio-visual media and mental health campaigns, the traditional manifestations of insanity are becoming increasingly offensive. They are more or less tolerated in the lower class, but this class is continually shrinking, while the middle class is growing. The new middle-class citizen tends to hide his disturbances where they will be least noticeable, in his soma. In so doing he kills two birds with one stone: not only does he conceal his disturbance, but by his paralysis, cardiac spasms, stomach ulcers, vomiting attacks, etc., he can gain attention from other people more easily and manipulate them with greater authority. Psychosomatic disorders in our society are manifestations of the triumph of medicine as a rational science. They indicate one of the directions the process of morbid secularization can take. Their meaning is the opposite to that which they held for primitive man: they denote a shrinking of the realm of the sacred.

From this point of view, two facts seem of great significance. When the author was studying the dreams of coloured people in Brazil in an area of acculturation and industrialization, he was struck by the fact that these dreams made increasing use of mechanical symbols instead of religious ones, reflecting the growth of industrialization. The human body (or the fears associated with it) were represented less by cosmic images such as water or the twin than by disrupted factories, broken tools, machines that were out of order, etc. The body had been rethought in unison with the ascendant mechanical society. Dream images had severed their links with the myths of the Creation; they had lost touch with the realm of the sacred. The second fact is that no two clinical pictures are more alike than that of the capitalist U.S.A. and that of communist Russia, in spite of the difference in ideologies. This is because underneath the antagonistic superstructures lie exactly the same realities of industrial society. Raymond Aron's demonstration of the genuine similarities between the two countries by an analysis of their representative economies can be extended, in our opinion, to the manifestations of morbidity. In Russia, where atheism is an openly professed communist dogma, there must necessarily be a rejection of anything that vaguely recalls the 'sacred disease'. Even psychosomatic disturbance carries a faint odour of idealism; therefore somatization will be built up to a maximum. (Neurotics have not disappeared in Russia, but are found in general hospitals.) In the U.S.A. religion has become no more than a Sunday activity. American psychiatrists recognize that the neuroses have changed shape in the last two decades, evolving towards organic manifestations, the only neuroses worthy of a middle-class society (where even the manual worker has changed classes in his own eyes, according to the results of surveys).

4   The formal laws

The world of the insane feeds on images and signs borrowed from the surrounding world. It does, of course, change their meaning, so that the image or the sign expresses an original personal experience rather than a commonplace experience neutralized by everyday forms of communication. But it preserves the formal laws—the principal ones at least—of the normal world. The study of these formal laws is still in its infancy. At the St Anne Hospital in Paris a group of linguists, psychologists and psychiatrists are conducting a study of the language of aphasics without reference to clinical classifications, the sample of terms merely being subjected to a frequency analysis.[31] It could be regretted that they have chosen a disorder caused by brain damage (disturbed cybernetics) rather than the language of schizophrenics (reoriented cybernetics). But it is a beginning. In fact, projects of this type ought not to remain on a statistical level and merely deal with the distribution of words in the formation of verbal sequences. They ought to take a structural approach which would concern itself with the nature and classification of words, and a topological approach which would deal with the transformation of words in relation to their existence in the original basic verbal space.

However, the few comments we made in the preceding paragraph are sufficient to show our essential point: the world of madness is part of the total system; it is always possible, by making the appropriate transformations, to link it with the total system. We still need to demonstrate that the reverse is true—in other words, that the system of what we call the 'normal mind' is an integral part of the world of madness. Some psychiatrists have, of course, retained the bipolar conception of the normal and the pathological; most of them, however, place between the two poles those entities which Grasset of Montpellier called 'half-mad' and 'half-rational'. On this basis it is possible to establish a whole topographical system, with genuine phenomena of contact, assimilation (morbid contagion) and acculturation. It would be a truly descriptive topography, one that eliminates value-judgments (in fact, at the same period as Grasset a discussion was taking place about the relation between genius and madness (Moreau of Tours, Lombroso) and sainthood and madness (Delacroix, Blondel)).

Today we know that we all carry within us the abyss that can swallow up our sanity (as defined by social consensus). Madness represents the emergence of deep-seated tendencies present in all human beings; alternatively, it is the disruptive factor in our personality which we look upon as a temptation both feared and desired and against which we build up defence systems and mechanisms of control. In short, we feel within us the stirrings of the dark side of our being. Naturally enough, it is the writer, who is more interested in the inner life than ordinary men, who has tended to emphasize this shadowy half of the personality, but he is only highlighting a constant. Stevenson symbolized it in the characters of Dr Jekyll and Mr Hyde. Conrad's character Leggatt, the murderer in *The Secret Sharer*, represents the outlaw and nightly companion of the captain who narrates the story and who feels linked with him in a mysterious bond of fellowship. Pirandello, in *Ciascuno a suo Modo*, speaks of the 'illegitimate thoughts, like bastard sons' who, 'far from the honest conjugal hearth of the conscience', allow us to entertain illicit relations with the world of madness in the vaults and caverns of our dwelling-place. It would even be possible to trace, in the work of these writers, a sociology of these illicit relations; they are especially manifest in periods of transition—in other words, of value-crisis (*Don Quixote*)—or in journey situations where contact is made with exotic lands and where the control of 'civilization' is removed or partly relaxed (Conrad).

We are thus able to experience, from the inside, a realm which we regard as totally foreign to our reason. Durkheim and Mauss's words about the primitive mentality could well be applied here: 'It is far from being the case that this mentality has no connection with our own. Of course, the terms that we unite in this way are not those that the Aborigine brings together; we choose them by other criteria and for other reasons; but the process itself by which the mind relates them does not differ essentially.' Or we could quote Lévi-Strauss's comments on Bergson and Rousseau in relation to totemism: 'They demonstrate that every human mind is a locus of virtual experience where what goes on in the minds of man, however remote they may be, can be investigated.'[32]

These two passages indicate no doubt an exorcizing of affectivity, whereas affectivity has a predominant place in morbid structures. 'The schizophrenic and primitive man,' says Bursztyn, 'do not classify objects, but their own representation of objects. The criterion they use does not derive from the object to be evaluated, but expresses the subject's point of view.'[33] Nevertheless, we can state (1) that classification is a logical operation obeying the same formal laws in the insane as in the sane person, (2) that we classify objects not so much according to their nature as according to the representation society has of these objects, so that the distinction is really one of degree, and (3) that even though it is necessary to bring in the 'subject's point of view' in schizophrenia, we can, for both affective structures and mental structures, discover within ourselves the laws of their disorganization or the principles of their morbid transformation.

The problem of the insane in society is not only the sick person's problem, but also the problem of the community. The sick person establishes a *modus vivendi* with his environment, and reciprocally the community tolerates certain forms of eccentricity, and dictates to the psychiatrist not so much the cure of the patient as the re-formulation of 'untamed' symptoms in an acceptable form.[34] Just as the previous chapter led us from social systems to systems of representations, the present chapter leads us from systems of representations to social systems. Intrapsychic phenomena are crystallized into social relations. The madman is to a certain extent the expression of our guilty conscience; he represents the chaotic part of ourselves that we wish to negate, exteriorized and operating in public. This is why we look upon him as an 'outlaw', a 'threat' to society. Our judgment of him is only the reflection or, more accurately, the projection, of the judgment we are making of a part of ourselves. Therefore madness has a social function in the same sense that crime, for Durkheim, has a social function. It enables us to free ourselves by transferring to others the dangers that threaten us. The madman may bear within him the human condition, but normal man is the seed-bed in which madness takes root.

219

5 Concluding remarks

We have attempted to show that the isolation of the insane and the private character of their symbolic activity are only one aspect of mental disorder, and not the most important aspect if we are to go beyond the superficial level. We have tried to bridge the gap between the mentally ill and society. The crises of the mind reflect influence either of the crises of society or of crises in the family within which the delusions or depression of the adult are shaped. The traumas or contradictions of religious, ethnic or economic groups, even if they are not considered causes of disorder, introduce themselves into psychic mechanisms and disturb their functioning. The neurotic and the psychotic do not remain unaffected, any more than the sane person, by these subtle, unconscious influences, these pressures or constraints from the environment. But what is more important, even if we do not accept admission to a mental hospital as the sole criterion of mental illness, as some authors have done, we have become aware that the definition of madness is always a social phenomenon; it varies according to place and time. The collectivity establishes the distinction between normal and pathological in accordance with its dominant values. (We mentioned the changing criteria of this differentiation: 'adjustment' under stable industrial capitalism, and 'the ability to define one's own norms' in our contemporary society of intensive production, where occupational and geographical mobility have become increasingly important.)

Finally, we tried to sketch, in the structuralist part of this work, the basic elements of a global 'social system' within which 'insanity' can be located, at the cleavages between subsystems or in marginal zones. It is always necessary to consider the total structure: the behaviour of the sick person affects the social units to which he belongs and, reciprocally, the characteristic structure of these units determines the responses of the sick person (isolation, rebellion, agitation, etc.).[35]

We have even tried to establish that the communication networks continue in spite of the interferences and especially in spite of our wish to appear 'other' than the insane (cf. Descartes's arrogant exclamation: '*Mais quoi, ce sont des fous!*'). In short, we believe we have succeeded, by drawing together all these statements, aetiological or structural, statistical or qualitative, in proving that insanity is essentially a social phenomenon and that it can be studied just as appropriately by sociological as by psychological analysis.

Notes

Introduction

1 *Culture, a Critical Review of Concepts and Definitions*, New York, 1963.
2 E.g. E. M. GRUENBERG and S. S. BELLIN, 'The Impact of Mental Disease on Society', in A. H. Leighton, J. A. Clausen and R. N. Wilson, eds., *Explorations in Social Psychiatry*, New York, 1957.
3 H. M. ADLER, 'The Relation between Psychiatry and Social Science', *Amer. J. Psychiat.*, vi (1927).
4 S. W. HARTWELL, 'Social Psychiatry, Our Task or a New Profession?' *ibid.*, xix (1940).
5 MAXWELL JONES, *Social Psychiatry, a Study of Therapeutic Communities*, Tavistock Publications, 1952.
6 M. K. OPLER, 'Social Psychiatry, Evolutionary, Existentialist and Transcultural Findings', *Psychosomatics*, ii (1961), 6, pp. 430–5.
7 H. S. SULLIVAN, 'Psychiatry: Introduction to the Study of Interpersonal Relations', *Psychiatry*, i (1938), pp. 121–34.
8 MASSERMAN, *Principles of Dynamic Psychiatry*, Philadelphia, 1946.
9 M. K. OPLER, *Culture, Psychiatry and Human Values*, Springfield, Illinois, 1956.
10 R. E. L. FARIS and H. W. DUNHAM, *Mental Disorders in Urban Areas*, Chicago, 1939.
11 G. DEVEREUX, *Reality and Dream: the Psychopathology of a Plains Indian*, New York, 1951.
12 DOLLARD, MILLER, DOOB, MOWRER and SEARS, *Frustration and Aggression*, New Haven, 1961.
13 J. P. VALABREGA, *La Relation Thérapeutique*, Flammarion, 1962.
14 H. BARUK, *La Psychiatrie Sociale*, P.U.F., Coll. 'Que Sais-je?', 669, 1955.
15 GABRIEL DESHAIES, *Psychopathologie générale*, P.U.F., 1959, p. 180.
16 T. D. ELIOT, in A. M. Rose, ed., *Mental Health and Mental Disorder, a Sociological Approach*, New York, 1955, and 'A Psychoanalytic Interpretation of Group Formation and Behavior', *Amer. J. Sociol.*, xxvi (1920).
17 H. BARUK, *op. cit.*
18 HANS STROTZKA, 'Sozialpsychiatrische Überlegungen', *Kölner Zeitsch. f. Soziol. und Sozialpsych.*, iii, Köln (1958).

221

19 A. M. ROSE, ed., *Mental Health and Mental Disorder, a Sociological Approach*, New York, 1955.
20 *J. Abnorm. Soc. Psychol.*, xxviii (1933).
21 L. L. BERNARD, *Social Psychology*, 1926 (ch. 13).
22 O. KLINEBERG, *Introduction to Social Psychology*, Sao Paulo, 1946.
23 G. DEVEREUX, *Mohave Ethnopsychiatry and Suicide*, Washington, 1961.
24 T. D. ELIOT, *op. cit.*

Chapter I The formation and development of a sociology of mental disorder

1 Passage quoted in footnote by J. Lacroix, *La Sociologie d'Auguste Comte*, P.U.F., 1956, p. 83.
2 *Cours de Philosophie Positive* (from vol. IV); *Discours sur l'Esprit Positif*, 1844; *Catéchisme Positiviste*, 1849.
3 C. BLONDEL, *La Conscience Morbide*, Alcan, 1914, p. 247.
4 PIERRE JANET, *L'Evolution Psychologique de la Personalité*, Maloine, 1929, and 'La Tension Psychologique et ses Oscillations' in *Traité de Psychologie* by Dumas, Alcan, 1923.
5 PIERRE JANET, *De l'Angoisse à l'Extase*, vol. I, Alcan, 1926.
6 LE GUILLANT, 'Introduction à une Psychopathologie sociale', *Evolution Psychiatrique*, i (1954), pp. 1–52.
7 JOSEPH GABEL, *La Réification*, Editions de Minuit, 1962, p. 235.
8 JOSEPH WORTIS, *Psychiatrie Soviétique*, P.U.F., 1953.
9 GABEL, *op. cit.*
10 *Ibid.*, p. 73.
11 R. BASTIDE, *Sociologie et Psychanalyse*, P.U.F., 1950.
12 *Ibid.*, pp. 90–5.
13 R. BASTIDE, 'Sociologie et psychanalyse', in *Traité de Sociologie*, by G. Gurvitch, vol. II, P.U.F., 1960, pp. 406–8.
14 E. V. SCHNEIDER, 'Sociological Concepts and Psychiatric Research', in *Interrelations between the Social Environment and Psychiatric Disorders*, Milbank Memorial Fund, New York, 1953.
15 Cf. the chapter by L. S. KUBIE in A. H. Leighton, J. A. Clausen and R. N. Wilson, eds., *Explorations in Social Psychiatry*, Basic Books, New York, 1952.
16 MORENO, 'The Concept of Sociodrama', *Psychodrama Monograph*, No. 1, Beacon House, 1943.
17 M. and MME VAN BOCKSTAELE, *Sociométrie*. . . .
18 MARVIN K. OPLER, *Culture, Psychiatry and Human Values*, Springfield, Ill., 1956.
19 ARNOLD M. ROSE, ed., *Mental Health and Mental Disorders: a Sociological Approach*, New York, 1955 (chapter by T. D. Eliot).
20 Cf. in the same work R. A. Schermerhorn's article.
21 P.U.F., 1952.
22 N. CAMERON, *The Psychology of Behavior Disorders: a Biosocial Interpretation*, Boston, 1947.
23 KAREN HORNEY, *The Neurotic Personality of Our Time*, New York, 1937.
24 T. M. NEWCOMB, *Social Psychiatry*, New York, 1950.
25 MME ROCHEBLAVE-SPENLÉ, *op. cit.*, p. 335.
26 ALEXANDER H. LEIGHTON, *My Name is Legion*, New York, 1959.
27 HARRY STACK SULLIVAN, 'Psychiatry: Introduction to the Study of Interpersonal Relations', *Psychiatry*, i (1938), pp. 121, 134; 'Conceptions of

Modern Psychiatry', *ibid.* (1940), pp. 1–117; 'A Note in the Implications of Psychiatry for Investigations in the Social Sciences', *Amer. J. Sociol.* (1937), pp. 848–61, etc.

28 A collection of the contributions to social psychiatry of a few of the members of this school may be found in Patrick Mullahy, ed., *A Study of Interpersonal Relations*, New York, 1949.

29 We refer in particular to the introduction by Bourricaud to the French translation of Talcott Parsons, *Eléments pour une Sociologie de l'Action*, Plon, 1955, and to ch. 5 of the same work. We also made much use of Parsons' contribution in *Interrelations between the Social Environment and Psychiatric Disorders*, Milbank Memorial Fund, New York, 1953.

30 PARSONS, *op. cit.*, p. 253.

31 This is the point of view defended by Zillborg in 'Psychiatry as a Social Science', *Amer. J. Psychiat.*, xcix (1943), pp. 585–8.

Chapter II Methodological problems

1 This paragraph summarizes a certain number of ideas developed by François Meyer, *Problématique de l'Evolution*, P.U.F., 1954, and Durkheim, *Le Suicide*, Alcan, 1897. Robinson ('Ecological Correlations and the Behavior of Individuals', *Amer. Sociol. Rev.*, 1950, pp. 351–7) criticizes the statistical method by demonstrating mathematically that it is not possible to infer individual correlations from sociological correlations; the properties of groups are not identical to the properties of individuals. We do no disagree, but merely think that Robinson should conclude that the sociology of mental disorder is not the same as social psychiatry; each field has its own methods.

2 We have made use in this section of an excellent mimeographed study by Victor D. Sanua, *The Epidemiology and Etiology of Mental Illness and Problems of Methodology . . . a Review of the Literature*, Yeshiva Univ., New York, s.d.

3 KRAEPELIN, *Psychiatrie*, Leipzig, 1909.

4 A good example of this may be found in Sanua, *op. cit.*, p. 44: the morbidity rates of various mental disorders in Baltimore and Tennessee are not comparable, owing to differences in methods of data-collection.

5 E.g. H. B. MURRAY, E. D. WITTKOWER, J. FRIED, H. ELLENBERGER, 'A Cross-Cultural Survey of Schizophrenic Symptomatology', *Int. J. Soc. Psychiat.*, ix, 4 (1963).

6 Cf. ODEGAARD, 'Emigration and Insanity', *Acta Psychiat. et Neurol.*, Suppl. 4, Copenhagen, 1932.

7 REMA LAPOUSSE, MARY A. MONK and MILTON TERRIS, 'The Drift Hypothesis and Socioeconomic Differentials in Schizophrenia', *Amer. J. Public Health*, xlvi (1956), p. 978–86.

8 Discussion in SCHERMERHORN, 'Social Psychiatry' in A. M. Rose, ed., *Mental Health and Mental Disorders, op. cit.*

9 H. B. ADAMS, 'Are Mental Hospital Admission Rates a Valid Measure of the Incidence of Mental Illness in the General Population?', 1957, quoted by Sanua, *op. cit.*

10 H. GOLDHAMER and A. MARSHALL, *Psychosis and Civilization: Two Studies in the Frequency of Mental Illness*, Glencoe, Ill., 1953.

11 Paper given by R. M. Wintrob at the author's seminar on social psychiatry.

12 However, Gartly E. Jaco, whose data we use here, does not think differences in attitudes are sufficient to explain this phenomenon:

'Mental Health of the Spanish-American in Texas', in M. K. Opler, ed., *Culture and Mental Health*, New York, 1959, pp. 467–85.

13 CARL BRUGGER, 'Versuch einer Geisteskrankenzahlung', in Thuringen, *Zeitsch. Ges. Neurol. und Psychiat.*, 133, 1931, pp. 352–91, and Erik Stromgren, 'Beitrag zur psychiatrischen Erblehre', *Acta Psychiat. et Neurol.*, Suppl. 19, 1938.

14 SANUA, *op. cit.*, p. 16.

15 K. H. FREMMING, 'The Expectation of Mental Uniformity in a Sample of the Danish Population', summarized by Sanua, *op. cit.*, p. 30.

16 R. W. HYDE, L. V. KINGSLEY and R. M. CHISHOLM, 'Study in Medical Sociology, III', *New England J. Med.*, xxi (1944), pp. 612–18.

17 JOSEPH W. EATON and ROBERT J. WEIL, *Culture and Mental Disorders*, Glencoe, Ill., 1955, particularly the chapters on methodology.

18 AUGUST B. HOLLINGSHEAD and FREDERICK G. REDLICH, *Social Class and Mental Illness: a Community Study*, New York, 1958.

19 V. D. SANUA, *op. cit.*, p. 26.

20 HOLLINGSHEAD and REDLICH, *op. cit.*

21 For a model of this type of questionnaire see T. G. Andrews, *Méthodes de la Psychologie* (French translation), II, P.U.F., 1952, pp. 706–10.

22 Cf. the discussion in Leighton, 'What is a Case?'—that is, how does one define a sick person?—in *Interrelations between the Social Environment and Psychiatric Disorders*, Milbank Memorial Fund, New York, 1953.

23 JASPERS, *Psychopathologie générale*, French translation, 1953; quoted by H. Duchêne, Le Mappian and Y. Roumagon, 'Influence du Milieu', *Psychiatrie*, ii (1955).

24 The bibliography on this question is vast; see in particular G. W. Allport, *The Use of Personal Documents in Psychological Science*, New York, 1942, L. Gottschalk, *The Use of Personal Documents in History, Anthropology and Sociology*, New York, 1945, and, for a condensed study of the problem, P. B. Foreman, 'The Theory of Case Studies', *Social Forces*, xxvi, 4 (1948).

25 W. H. SEWELL, 'Infant Training and the Personality of the Child', in A. M. Rose, *op. cit.*

26 S. ARIETI, *Interpretation of Schizophrenia*, New York, 1955.

27 See below, ch. 4. On the dialectic between the case history and ecology, see Robert E. L. Faris, in J. McV. Hunt, ed., *Personality and the Behavior Disorders*, New York, 1944.

28 V. D. SANUA, 'Comparison of Jewish and Protestant Paranoid and Catatonic Patients', *Dis. Nerv. Syst.*, xxvi, 6 (1962) (1–7).

29 On ethnopsychiatry, see R. Bastide, 'Ethnologie et Psychiatrie', in Poirier, *Traité d'Ethnologie*, Gallimard; and, on the comparative method, see John W. M. Whieting, 'The Cross-cultural Method', in Gordner Lindsey, ed., *Handbook of Social Psychology*.

30 R. BASTIDE, *Sociologie et Psychanalyse*, P.U.F., 1950, ch. 8.

31 Quoted by M. K. OPLER, *op. cit.*

32 Cf. A. H. LEIGHTON, T. A. LAMBO, C. C. HUGHES, D. C. LEIGHTON, J. M. MURPHY and D. B. MACKLIN, *Psychiatric Disorders among the Yoruba*, Cornell Univ. Press, 1963.

33. A. KARDINER, *The Individual and His Society*, New York, 1939.

34 A. B. HOLLINGSHEAD and F. C. REDLICH, *Social Class and Mental Illness*, New York, 1950.

35 BACHELARD, *Le Rationalisme Appliqué*, P.U.F., 1949, ch. 3.

36 E.g. COURCHET and MAUCORPS in their study of the 'social vacuum', *Le Vide Social*, Mouton et Cie., The Hague.

37 DAVID AZOUBEL NETO, 'Localizaçao em Psicoterapia do Groupo', *Rev. de Psich. Normal e Patologica*, São Paulo, Brazil, iii, 3, 4 (1957).
38 ASYA L. KADIS and C. WINICK, 'The Role of the Deviant in the Therapy of Group', *Int. J. Soc. Psychiat.*, vi, 3–4 (1960).
39 COURCHET and MAUCORPS, *op. cit.*

Chapter III   Prolegomena to a sociology of mental disorder

1 Discussed, for example, in DOUGLAS G. HARING, ed., *Personal Character and Cultural Milieu*, Syracuse Univ. Press, 1949. See also R. Benedict, *Patterns of Culture*, Boston, 1934, and ch. 23 (by Gregory Bateson) in McV. Hunt, ed., *Personality and the Behavior Disorders*, vol. II, New York, 1944.
2 JOHN P. FOLEY, JR., 'The Criterion of Abnormality', *J. Abnorm. Soc. Psychol.*, xxx, 3.
3 MARIE JAHODA, in Arnold M. Rose, ed., *Mental Health and Mental Disorder*, New York, 1955.
4 HENRY G. WEGROCKI, 'A Critique of Cultural and Statistical Concepts of Abnormality', in C. Kluckhohn and H. A. Murray, *Personality in Nature, Society and Culture*, New York, 1948.
5 FRANCIS L. K. HSU, 'Anthropology and Psychiatry: a Definition of Objectives and Their Implications', *Southwestern J. Anthrop.*, viii, 2 (1952).
6 See, for example, Y. Roumejon, 'Le Problème de l'Identité des Psychoses à travers les Facteurs ethniques', *Evol. Psychiat.*, iii (1956).
7 J. J. B. MORGAN, *The Psychology of Abnormal People*, New York, 1928.
8 G. Kluckhohn quoted by Marie Jahoda, 'Environment and Mental Health', *Int. Soc. Sci. J.* (English version) Unesco, xi, 1 (1959).
9 RALPH LINTON, *Culture and Mental Disorders*, Springfield, Ill., 1956.
10 R. M. and C. H. BERNDT, 'The Concept of Abnormality in an Australian Aboriginal Society', in G. B. Wilbur and W. Muensterberger, *Psychoanalysis and Culture*, New York, 1951.
11 The bibliography on this subject is never-ending. It can be found in Linton, *op. cit.* The example of Buddhism was taken from Dubois, 'Some Anthropological Perspectives on Psychoanalysis', *Psychoanal. Rev.*, xxiv (1937), and one particular idea from George de Vos, 'A Quantitative Rorschach Assessment of Maladjustment and Rigidity in Acculturating Japanese Americans', *Genetic. Psych. Mon.*, lii (1955). A good summary of present-day thinking on this subject may be found in Henri Ellenberger, 'Aspects culturels de la maladie mentale', *Rev. de Psycho. des Peuples.*, xv, 3.
12 JOHN J. HONIGMAN, 'Toward a distinction between psychiatric and social abnormality, *Soc. Forces*, xxxi.
13 GEORGE DEVEREUX, 'Normal and Abnormal, the Key Problem in Psychiatric Anthropology', *Anthrop. Soc. of Washington*, 1956.
14 KURT GOLDSTEIN, *The Structure of the Organism*, French tr., Gallimard, 1951.
15 G. CANGUILHEM, *Essais sur quelques Problèmes concernant le Normal et le Pathologique*, Publ. Fac. des Lettres de Strasbourg, 1950.
16 M. JAHODA, *op. cit.*
17 A confirmation that sex operates solely as a sociological category is that in Africa also, wherever data are available, there is a predominance of men over women (1·5–1·7 men to 1 woman).
18 BENJAMIN MALZBERG, *Social and Biological Aspects of Mental Disease*, New York, 1940.

19 M. E. LINDEN and D. COURTNEY, 'The Human Life Cycle and Its Inter-
ruptions', in A. M. Rose, ed., *Mental Health and Mental Disorder, a
Sociological Approach*, New York, 1955.

20 J. C. CAROTHERS, *The African Mind in Health and Disease*, World Health
Organization, Geneva, 1953.

21 Cf. H. DUCHÊNE, 'Parts respectives de l'Hérédité, de la Constitution et
du Milieu dans la Pathologie des Troubles Mentaux', *Psychiatrie*, 2,
1955.

22 H. DUCHÊNE, *op. cit.*; V. D. SANUA, *The Epidemiology and Etiology of
Mental Illness: a Methodological Study*, Yeshiva Univ., New York, s.d.;
FRANK KALLMAN, 'The Genetic Theory of Schizophrenia', *Amer. J.
Psychiat.*, 1946; D. JACKSON, 'A Critique of the Literature on the
Genetics of Schizophrenia', in *Etiology of Schizophrenia*, New York,
1960.

23 GLASS, quoted by J. W. Eaton and R. J. Weil, *Culture and Mental
Disorders*, Glencoe, Ill., 1955.

24 V. D. SANUA, *op. cit.*

25 In addition to H. EY, *Etudes Psychiatriques*, vol. I, Desclée de Brouwer,
1948, cf. in particular L. Bonnafé, H. Ey, S. Follin, J. Lacan and J.
Rouart, *Le Problème de la Psychogenèse des Névroses et des Psychoses*,
Desclée de Brouwer, 1950.

26 On the subject of this evolution cf. R. Bastide, *Sociologie et Psychanalyse*. Also E. Fromm, 'Individual and Social Origins of Neurosis', in
A. M. Rose, *op. cit.*, and the study by L. S. Kubin on the relation between social forces and neurotic processes in A. H. Leighton, J. A.
Clausen, R. N. Wilson, *et al.*, *Explorations in Social Psychiatry*, New
York, 1957; also Karl Birnbaum, *Sociologie der Neurosen*, Berlin,
1933.

27 H. GOLDHAMER and A. MARSHALL, *Psychosis and Civilization: Two Studies
in the Frequency of Mental Illness*, Glencoe, Ill., 1953.

28 On the relation between organic disorders and sociocultural factors, see,
for example, Alexander H. Leighton, *My Name is Legion*, New York,
1959.

29 We quoted Le Guillant above. Similar ideas can be found in France in
the work of Follin as well as in Bonnafé, Ey, Follin, Lacan and Rouart,
op. cit.; and, in the United States, Kingsley Davis, 'Mental Hygiene and
the Class Structure', *Psychiatry*, 1938, pp. 56–65.

30 On the conflict between various conceptions of social influences in the
pathogenesis of mental illness, besides the authors already quoted in
the notes to this chapter, see M. K. Opler, *Culture, Psychiatry and
Human Values*, Springfield, Ill., 1956.

31 In this historical survey we have especially made use of the work of
Delay, Deniker, Pichot, Mlle Lemperière and Sadoun, 'Délires à Deux
et à Plusieurs: Étude clinique de Vingt-deux Familles délirantes', *Congrès Aliénistes et Neurologistes* (Nice), Coueslant, Cahors, 1955. Interesting statistics can be found in A. Gralnick, '*Folie à Deux*, the
Psychosis of Association: A Review of 103 cases and the Entire English
Literature', *Psychiat. Quart.*, 16 (1942):

Relationship	No. of combinations	No. of people
Husband-wife	11	22
Wife-husband	15	30
2 sisters	35	70
2 sisters (twins)	5	10
3 sisters	5	15
2 brothers	10	20
2 brothers (twins)	3	6
3 brothers	1	3
Sister-brother	4	8
Brother-sister	2	4
Mother-daughter	16	32
Father-daughter	1	2
Mother-son	8	16
Father-son	1	2
Patient-patient	4	8
Friend-friend	5	10

32 Even in cases of mother-child or father-child psychosis, the concept of a 'joint unconscious' developing in two people living in a close symbiotic relationship may in fact be a more heuristic notion than the notion of hereditary transmission.

33 HEUYER, 'Les Psychoses Collectives', *Rev. du Praticien*, v. 15 (1955).

34 JOHN DOLLARD and N. E. MILLER, *Personality and Psychotherapy: an Analysis in terms of Learning, Thinking, Culture*, New York, 1956.

35 R. BASTIDE, *Sociologie et Psychanalyse*, P.U.F., 1951.

36 Cf. G. DUMAS, 'Contagion mentale. Epidémies mentales. Folies collectives. Folies grégaires', *Rev. Philos.*, i (1916).

37 HAMON, 'Les Psychoses collectives', *Congrès des Médecins Aliénistes*, 55, *op. cit.*

38 H. D. LASSWELL, 'Propaganda and Mass Insecurity', *Psychiatry*, xiii (1950), pp. 283–99.

39 M. CERTEAU, in J. J. Surin, *Correspondance*, Desclée de Brouwer, 1966.

40 GABRIEL DESHAIES, *Psychopathologie Générale*, P.U.F., 1959, p. 180.

41 ERNESTO DE MARTINO, *La Terra del Rimorso*, Milan, 1961.

42 ERICH FROMM, *The Sane Society*, London, 1956.

43 G. DEVEREUX, 'Maladjustment and Social Neurosis', *Amer. Sociol. Rev.*, iv, 6 (1939).

44 READ BAIN, 'Sociology and Psychoanalysis', *Amer. Sociol. Rev.*, i (1936).

45 See also R. LAFORGUE, *Libido, Angst und Zivisation*, Vienna, 1932.

46 FRANZ ALEXANDER, 'Psychoanalysis and Social Disorganization', *Amer. J. Sociol.*, Vol. 42, 2nd Semester, 1937.

47 R. BASTIDE, *op. cit.*

Chapter IV From ecology to the study of communities

1 P. A. SOROKIN and C. C. ZIMMERMAN, *Principles of Rural-Urban Sociology*, New York, 1929, pp. 164–5; CLARENCE W. SCHRODER, 'Mental Disorders in Cities', *Amer. J. Sociol.*, xlviii, 1 (1942); B. MALZBERG, *Social and Biological Aspects of Mental Disease*, New York, 1940, ch. 3. On the other

hand, Deshaies in France finds no significant difference in numbers between the mentally ill of rural origin and those of urban origin (*Le Recensement des Psychopathies en France*, Imprimerie Contemporaine, 1938).

2 SIVADON, 'Géographie Humaine et Psychiatrie', *Annales Médico-psychologiques*, 106th year, 1948.

3 M. B. OWEN, 'Alternative Hypotheses for the Explanation of Faris and Dunham's Results', *Amer. J. Sociol.*, xlvii (1941), pp. 48–52; E. GARTLY JACO, 'Attitude Toward and Incidence of Mental Disorder', *Southwestern Soc. Science Quart.*, xxxviii (1957), pp. 27–38; O. ØDEGAARD, 'Current Studies of Incidence and Prevalence of Hospitalized Mental Patients in Scandinavia', in P. H. Hoch and J. Zubin, eds., *Comparative Epidemiology of the Mental Disorders*, New York, 1961.

4 TSUNG-YI LIN, 'A Study of the Incidence of Mental Disorders in Other Cultures', *Psychiatry*, xvi (1953), pp, 313–36.

5 Cf. A. LEIGHTON, J. A. CLAUSEN and R. N. WILSON, eds., *Explorations in Social Psychiatry*, New York, 1957 (E. Leacock's chapter).

6 V. D. SANUA, *The Epidemiology and Etiology of Mental Illness and Problems of Methodology*, Yeshiva Univ., New York, pp. 29–35.

7 *Ibid.*, pp. 44–5.

8 PIERRE SCHERER, 'Les Psychoses en Milieu Rural', *Le Concours Médical*, colloque de psycho-sociologie agricole, Tours, 14 June 1959.

9 JOSEPH W. EATON and ROBERT J. WEIL, *Culture and Mental Disorders: a Comparative Study of the Hutterites and Other Populations*, Glencoe, Ill., 1955; BERT KAPLAN and THOMAS F. A. PLAUT, *Personality in a Communal Society: an Analysis of the Mental Health of the Hutterites*, Univ. of Kansas, 1956.

10 HARVEY ZORBAUGH, *The Gold Coast and the Slum*, Chicago, 1929; N. ANDERSON, *The Hobo*, Chicago, 1923; BURGESS, *The Urban Community*, Chicago, 1926; C. R. SHAW, *Delinquency Areas*, Chicago, 1929; RECKLESS, *Vice in Chicago*, Chicago, 1933; E. R. MOWRER, *The Family, Its Organization and Disorganization*, Chicago, 1932, etc.

11 ROBERT E. L. FARIS and H. WARREN DUNHAM, *Mental Disorders in Urban Areas*, Chicago, 1934.

12 F. A. ROSS, 'Ecology and the Statistical Method', *Amer. J. Sociol.*, 1933.

13 E. MOWRER, *Disorganization, Personal and Social*, New York, 1942, chs. 15 and 16.

14 S. A. QUEEN, 'The Ecological Study of Mental Disorders', *Amer. Sociol. Rev.*, v (1940).

15 A. W. SCHRÖDER, *op. cit.*

16 In ch. 24 of J. MCV. HUNT, ed., *Personality and the Behavior Disorders*, Vol. II, New York, 1944.

17 W. L. J. DEE, 'An Ecological Study of Mental Disorders in Metropolitan St. Louis', thesis, Washington Univ., 1939.

18 S. A. QUEEN, *op. cit.*

19 'The Epidemiology of Mental Disorders in a Political-type City, 1946–1952', in *Interrelations between the Social Environment and Psychiatric Disorders*, Milbank Memorial Fund, New York, 1953. Cf. E. Gartly Jaco, *The Social Epidemiology of Mental Disorders, a Psychiatric Survey of Texas*, New York, 1960.

20 CHOMBART DE LAUWE, *Paris et l'Agglomération Parisienne*, 2 vols., P.U.F., 1952.

21 E. M. GRUENBERG, 'Community Conditions and Psychosis of the Elderly', *Amer. J. Psychiat.*, 1954.

22 FRANK A. ROSS, 'Ecology and the Statistical Method', *Amer. J. Sociol*, xxxviii (1933).

23 KROUT, 'A Note on Dunham's Contribution to the Ecology of Functional Psychosis', *Amer. Sociol. Rev.*, iii (1938).

24 E. GARTLY JACO, 'The Social Isolation Hypothesis and Schizophrenia', *Amer. Sociol. Rev.*, xix, 3 (1954), pp. 567–77.

25 Ch. 24 in MCV. HUNT, *op. cit.*

26 H. W. DUNHAM, 'The Social Personality of the Catatonic Schizophrene', *Amer. J. Sociol.*, xlix (1944), pp. 508–18.

27 M. L. KOHN and G. A. CLAUSEN, 'Social Isolation and Schizophrenia', *Amer. Sociol. Rev.*, xx, 3 (1955), pp. 265–73.

28 S. KIRSON WEINBERG, 'A Sociological Analysis of a Schizophrenic Type', *Amer. Sociol. Rev.*, xv, (1950), pp. 600–10.

29 'Personal Disorder and Spatial Mobility', *Amer. J. Sociol.*, 48 (1942).

30 RONALD FREEDMAN, *Recent Migration to Chicago*, 1950.

31 MARY H. LYSTAD, 'Social Mobility among Schizophrenic Patients', *Amer. Sociol. Rev.*, xxii, 3 (1957), pp. 288–99.

32 B. D. PAUL gave a good example of this in the case of Maria, a girl with a masculine personality who lived in a Guatemalan village, i.e. in an essentially patriarchal culture. He explains her psychiatric disturbance by the fact that Guatemalan women are expected to perform only one role (mother-faithful-wife-homemaker). He adds that in the United States she would have survived, as she could have chosen from the series of feminine roles offered by American society: mother, glamour-girl, business woman, etc. ('Mental Disorder and Self-regulating Processes in Culture, a Guatemalan Illustration', in *Interrelations between . . . , op. cit.*).

33 PAUL HALMOS, *Solitude and Privacy, a Study of Social Isolation, Its Causes and Therapy*, London, s.d.

Chapter V The psychiatry of the total society: from occupation and social class to the industrial society

1 FRANZ ALEXANDER, 'Psychoanalysis and Social Disorganization', *Amer. J. Sociol.*, xlii, 2nd Semester, 1937.

2 *Amer. Sociol. Rev.*, April 1947.

3 *Solitude and Privacy, a Study of Social Isolation, Its Causes and Therapy*, London, s.d.

4 L. STERN, *Kulturkreis und Form der geistigen Erkrankung*, Halle, 1913.

5 E. MIRA, 'Le Rôle des Conditions Sociales dans la Genèse des Troubles Mentaux', *IIᵉ Congrès Int. Hyg. Men.*, Paris, I, 1937. In France the occupational aspect of mental disorder has received a great deal of attention, all the way from A. Marie, *Travail et Folie: Influence Professionnelle sur l'Etiologie Pathologique*, Paris, 1909, to P. Sivadon and Lévy-Klein, 'Maturation Affective: Profession et Troubles Mentaux', *Ann. Médico-psycho.*, i, 1 (1951).

6 Mouton et Cie.

7 H. BARUK and J. GUILHOT, 'Essai sur le Rôle de la Psychiatrie Sociale dans le Développement des Sciences Administratives: la Cas des "Psychallergies Administratives"', *Ann. Médico-psycho.*, 120ᵉ année, i (1962), pp. 235–78.

8 IDA BERGER and R. BENJAMIN, 'Maladies Mentales et Profession,

Contribution à l'Étude Sociologique des Troubles Mentaux dans le Milieu des Enseignants', in *l'Univers des Instituteurs*, Editions de Minuit, 1964, pp. 174, 212.

9 BEN Z. LOCKE, M. KRAMER, C. TIMBERLAKE, E. PASAMANICK and D. SMELTZER, 'Problems in Interpretation of Patterns of First Admissions to Ohio State Public Mental Hospitals for Patients with Schizophrenic Reactions', *Psychol. Res. Rep.*, x (1958), pp. 172–96.

10 ROBERT M. FRUMKIN, 'Occupation and Major Mental Disorders', in A. M. Rose, *Mental Health and Mental Disorder*, New York, 1955.

11 Summary of Frumkin's chapter by V. D. SANUA, *The Epidemiology and Etiology of Mental Illness and Problems of Methodology*, Yeshiva Univ., New York, s.d., pp. 55, 56.

12 ROBERT E. CLARK, 'The Relationship of Schizophrenia to Occupational Income and Occupational Prestige', *Amer. Sociol. Rev.*, xiii (1948), pp. 325–30.

13 'Psychoses, Income and Occupational Prestige', in Bendix and Lipset, *Class, Status and Power*, Glencoe, Ill., 1953.

14 FRUMKIN, *op. cit.*

15 'Social Technique, Social Status and Social Change in Illness', in Kluckhohn and Murray, *Personality in Nature, Society and Culture*, New York, 1948.

16 CHRISTOPHER TIETZE, 'Epidemiology of Mental Disorders', *Milbank Memorial Fund*, 1950.

17 KAREN HORNEY, 'Inhibitions dans le Travail', *Psyché*, iv, 33 (1949), pp. 581–95.

18 J. LUCIEN BARA, 'Psychologie Industrielle', *Psyché*, v, 39 (1950), pp. 76–8.

19 MARTIN GILBERT, 'Accidents de Travail', *Psyché*, vi, 53 (1951), pp. 185–7.

20 In C. KLUCKHOHN and H. A. MURRAY, eds., *op. cit.*

21 T. A. C. RENNIE, L. SROLE, M. K. OPLER and T. S. LANGNER, 'Urban Life and Mental Health, Socioeconomic Status and Mental Disorder in the Metropolis', *Amer. J. Psychiat.*, cxiii (1957), pp. 831–7.

22 AUGUST B. HOLLINGSHEAD and FREDERICK C. REDLICH, *Social Class and Mental Illness, a Community Study*, New York, 1958.

23 J. K. MYERS and L. SCHAFFER, 'Social Stratification and Psychiatric Practice', *Amer. Sociol. Rev.*, xix, 3 (1954), pp. 307–10. Cf. also, by the same authors, 'Psychotherapy and Social Stratification', *Psychiatry*, xvii (1954).

24 SAXON GRAHAM, 'Socioeconomic Status and Illness and the Use of Medical Services', *Milbank Mem. Fund Quart.*, xxxv (1957).

25 KATHERINE B. LAUGHTON, 'Socioeconomic Status and Illness', *ibid.*, xxxvi (1958), pp. 46–57.

26 PAUL LEMKAU, CHRISTOPHER TIETZE and MARCIA COOPER, 'Mental Hygiene Problems in an Urban District', *Ment. Hygiene*, xxvi (1942).

27 B. KAPLAN, R. B. REED and W. RICHARDSON, 'A Comparison of the Incidence of Hospitalized and Non-hospitalized Cases of Psychosis in Two Communities', *Amer. Sociol. Rev.*, xxi (1951), pp. 472–9.

28 V. D. SANUA, *op. cit.*, pp. 61–3.

29 W. L. WARNER, 'Society, the Individual and His Mental Disorder', *Amer. J. Psychiat.*, xciv (1937); GREEN, 'The Middle-class Male Child and Neurosis', *Amer. Sociol. Rev.*, ii (1946), B. H. ROBERTS and J. K. MYERS, 'Schizophrenia in the Youngest Male Child of the Lower Middle Class', *Amer. J. Psych.*, cxii (1955).

30 'Social Mobility and Mental Illness', *Amer. Sociol. Rev.*, xix, 5 (1954),

pp. 577–84. See also E. Ellis, 'Social Psychological Correlates of Upward Social Mobility among Unmarried Career Women', *Amer. Sociol. Rev.*, xvii (1952), pp. 558–63.
31 MARY H. LYSTAD, 'Social Mobility among Schizophrenic Patients', *Amer. Sociol. Rev.*, xxii, 3 (1957), pp. 288–99.
32 S. L. MORRISSON, 'Principles and Methods of Epidemiological Research', *J. Ment. Sci.*, cv (1959), pp. 999–1011.
33 The source of information for this summary of Richard's theories is not his article in *L'Année Sociologique*, but a revised and supplemented version of it delivered as a lecture, which has remained unpublished, at Bordeaux University.
34 Cf., for example, N. J. Demerath's discussion of 'Schizophrenia among Primitives', in A. M. Rose, *Mental Health and Mental Disorder*, New York, 1955.
35 R. BASTIDE, 'Les Maladies Mentales des Noirs en Amérique du Sud', E. L. Margets, ed., *Psychiatrie Africaine.*
36 The main sociological source of material here is the work of Georges Friedmann and his followers and, from the psychiatric point of view, James S. Bossard, *Social Change and Social Problems*, New York, 2nd ed., 1938; Caudell, Redlich, Gilmore and Brody, 'Social Structure and Interaction Processes on a Psychiatric Ward', *Amer. J. Orthopsychiat.*, xxii (1952); Butler, 'Industrial Psychiatry', in *Symposium on Preventive and Social Psychiatry*, Washington, 1958; A. H. McLean and G. C. Taylor, *Mental Health in Industry*, New York, 1958.
37 *New Ways in Psychoanalysis*, New York, 1939.
38 M. MEAD, ed., *Sociétés, Traditions et Technologie*, U.N.E.S.C.O., 1953.
39 Some authors have justifiably reacted against the idea that industrialization is solely responsible for mental disorder in developing countries, in particular Geoffrey Tooth, *Studies in Mental Illness in the Gold Coast*, London, 1950, and Hollowell, 'Values, Acculturation and Mental Health', *Amer. J. Orthopsychiat.* xx (1950).
40 A good example of this is given by Devereux: the Mohave Indians in the U.S.A., who were prevented from expressing their aggressive tendencies in tribal warfare, did not repress these tendencies, but diverted them towards sexual success (*Mohave Ethnopsychiatry and Suicide*, Washington, 1961). On another level it has been universally noted by anthropologists that acculturation produces an increase in witchcraft, which acts as a compensation for neurosis.
41 CAROTHERS, *The African Mind in Health and Disease*, W.H.O., Geneva, 1953. The effects of industrialization are followed and supplemented by the effects of urbanization. Tsung-Yi Lin, 'Les Effets de l'Urbanisation sur la Santé Mentale', *Rev. Int. des Sc. Sociales*, U.N.E.S.C.O., xi, 1 (1959).
42 KAREN HORNEY, *The Neurotic Personality of Our Time*, New York, 1932. Cf. C. Kluckhohn, *Mirror for Man*, New York, 1949: 'The existing educational system ... is torn between conditioning children for the theoretically desirable co-operative objectives or to the existing competitive realities.'
43 M. MONTASSUT and C. LEROY, 'De Quelques Répercussions Psychologiques et Psychiatriques Contemporaines', *Gaz. Méd. France*, lxix (1962), pp. 1107–26.
44 YVES PÉLICIER, *Intégration des Données Sociologiques*, Masson et Cie., 1964. The effects of present-day working conditions on mental health have been the subject of important research by Dr Sivadon and Dr Veil

in France. From the sociological angle, see G. Friedmann, *Le Travail en Miettes*, p. 218 and pp. 333–4.

45 DUMAZEDIER, *Vers une Civilisation du Loisir*, 1962.

46 C. KLUCKHOHN, *op. cit.*, p. 291.

47 READ BAIN, 'Our Schizoid Culture', *Sociol. and Soc. Res.*, xix (1935).

48 A. and H. TORRUBIA, 'Contribution à Une Psychopathologie Sociale', *Inst. Nat. d'Hygiène*, Monographie No. 7 (1955); Y. Champion, *Migration et Maladie Mentale*, Arnette, Paris, 1958.

49 Thesis, Algiers, 1962.

50 J. M. SUTTER, quoted by Y. PÉLICIER, *op. cit.*, p. 189 (footnote).

51 G. GURVITCH, *La Vocation Actuelle de la Sociologie*, P.U.F., 1950, and *Traité de Sociologie*, P.U.F. 2 vols., 1958–60.

52 In the special issue of *Esprit*, 'Misère de la Psychiatrie', xx, 12 (1952). The idea of a psychological threshold, which, as we saw in our historical chapter, was important in Janet's work, appears here to be fundamental. Cf. J. Vie, 'A propos de l'Augmentation du Nombre des Aliénés, le Seuil de Résistance Psychique et les Difficultés de la Vie', *XVIIᵉ Congrès Int. d'Hyg Ment.*, i., (1937).

Chapter VI   The psychiatry of social groups: I. Religious groups

1 Quoted by H. DUCHÊNE, LE MAPPIAN and Y. ROUMAGON, 'Influence du Milieu', *Psychiatrie*, ii (1955). Jaspers, on the other hand, states that the incidence of mental disorder is lowest among Christians, higher among Jews and highest in Nonconformist sects; in other words, it increases as the religion becomes less individualistic and more collectivity-oriented. But in the case of the Jews the religious factor is linked with the influence of social discrimination, and Nonconformist sects tend to attract mentally-sick people rather than produce them (Karl Jaspers, *Psychopathology*). Consequently, Jaspers's statistics do not contradict Dayton's.

2 STONEQUIST, *The Marginal Man, a Study in Personality and Culture Conflict*, New York, 2nd Ed., 1961.

3 KLINEBERG, *Race Differences*, New York, 1935.

4 A more extensive discussion of these problems can be found in *Religion, Culture and Mental Health*, New York, 1961.

5 Quoted by HALÉVI; cf. note 10.

6 Rates per 100,000 population:

	Psychosis	Neurosis and personality disorders
Israelis	138·7	273·4
Immigrants from:		
Eastern Europe	124·3	160·2
The Balkans	144·6	180·8
Central Europe	137·7	191·6
Iraq	140·4	235·3
The Yemen	123·3	221·2
North Africa	140·2	254·5
Turkey	184·5	279·8
Iran	197·3	318·1

7 Quoted by YVES PÉLICIER, *Intégration des Données Sociologiques*, Masson et Cie., 1964, pp. 155–6.

8	Natives	Immigrants before 1948	Immigrants 1949–54	Immigrants after 1948
Psychosis	62·1	75·6	63·8	63·8
Neurosis	10·8	13·9	19·6	14·1
Mental deficiency	5·0	0·6	2·4	2·1
Personality disorders	22·1	9·9	14·2	20·0
	100·0	100·0	100·0	100·0

| 9 Diagnostic category | Rate per 100,000 population | | | |
	Towns	Villages	Co-operatives	Kibbutzim
Psychosis	91·3	100·8	70·3	90·8
Neurosis	20·9	25·5	12·6	24·0
Mental deficiency	2·9	2·0	2·4	2·5
Personality disorders	20·4	15·7	15·0	20·1
	135·5	144·0	100·3	137·4

10 H. S. HALÉVI, 'Frequency of Mental Illness among Jews in Israel', *Int. J. Soc. Psychiat.*, ix, 4 (1963).

11 L. SROLE, T. S. LANGUER, S. T. MICHEL, M. K. OPLER, T. A. C. RENNIE, eds., *Mental Health in the Metropolis: the Midtown Study*, Vol. I, New York, 1962.

12 A. B. HOLLINGSHEAD and F. C. REDLICH, *Social Class and Mental Illness, a Community Study*, New York, 1958.

13 P. BARRABEE and O. VAN MERING, 'Ethnic Variations in Mental Stress in Families with Psychotic Children', *Social Forces*, 1953, pp. 48–53.

14 K. MYERS and B. H. ROBERTS, *Family and Class Dynamics in Mental Illness*, New York, 1959.

15 V. D. SANUA, 'A Comprehensive Study of Schizophrenics of Different Backgrounds (Italian, Irish, Jews and Protestants)', mimeograph.

16 PAUL BERGMAN, 'A Religious Conversation in the Course of Psychotherapy', *Amer. J. Psychotherapy*, vii, 1 (1953).

17 *Amer. J. Psychiat.*, i (1944).

18 VIKTOR FRANKL, *Aetzliche Seelsorg*, Vienna, 1946.

19 SIMON DOMINGER, ed., *Religion and Human Behavior*, New York, 1954. In the city the number of cases where religion plays no part either directly or indirectly is naturally higher (Samuel Southard, quoted by Oates).

20 WAYNE E. OATES, *Religious Factors in Mental Illness*, New York, 1955.

21 J. W. EATON and R. J. WEIL, *Culture and Mental Illness: a Community Study*, New York, 1958.

22 P. CHOMBART DE LAUWE, 'La Maladie Mentale comme Phénomène Social', *Inst. Nat. d'Hygiène*, Monographie No. 7, Paris, 1955; M. COLINON, *Faux*

Prophètes et Sectes d'Aujourd'hui, Plon, 1953; DELAY PICHOT, BRISSON, etc., 'Etude d'un Groupe d'Adeptes d'Une Secte Religieuse', *Encéphale*.
23 *Op. cit.*
24 J. G. MCKENZIE, *Nervous Disorders and Religion*, London, 1951.

Chapter VII   The psychiatry of social groups: II. Ethnic groups

1 We have omitted the whole question of the Negro, to which we intend to devote a separate book in collaboration with Dr Raveau.
2 OTTO KLINEBERG, *Race Differences*, New York, 1935.
3 STONEQUIST, *The Marginal Man: a Study in Personality and Culture Conflict*, New York, 2nd ed., 1961.
4 HENRY PRATT FAIRCHILD, *Immigration*, New York, 1913.
5 This paragraph summarizes the criticisms of B. Malzberg in Benjamin Malzberg and Everett S. Lee, *Migration and Mental Disease*, New York, 1956, ch. 6.
6 ORNUEV ØDEGAARD, 'Emigration and Insanity', *Acta Psychiat. et Neurol.*, Scand. Suppl., iv (1932), and 'The Distribution of Mental Disease in Norway', *ibid.*, xx (1945).
7 MALZBERG and LEE, *op. cit.*
8 MARTIN H. KEELER and MINTAUTS VITOLS, *Migration and Schizophrenia in North Carolina Negroes*, quoted by V. D. Sanua, *The Epidemiology and Ætiology of Mental Illness and Problems of Methodology*, Yeshiva Univ., New York, s.d.
9 From the sociological point of view, the work of Stoetzel and Girard and that of Liepvre and Bousquet, published by the Institut National des Etudes Démographiques, provide a framework which should be compulsory for future psychiatric research. Among the numerous studies by psychiatrists, see C. F. Darlet, 'Les Psychopathes Etrangers à l'Hôpital Henri-Rousselle', thesis, 1920; G. Boitelle and C. Boitelle-Lentulo, 'Psychoses réactionelles au Dépaysement des Travailleurs Étrangers', *XLVIIᵉ Congrès Méd. et Neur.*, Clermont-Ferrand, 1949, and *IIᵉ Congrès*, Luxemburg, 1952; J. Cohen, 'La Santé Mentale chez les Sujets Transplantés en sans Foyer', *Bull. Féd. Mond. pour la Santé Mentale*, August 1950; Gilon, H. Duchêne and Y. Champion, 'Pathologie Mentale de la Mobilité Géographique', *Encylopédie Médico-Chirurgicale, Psychiatrie*; Y. Champion, *Migration et Maladie Mentale*, Arnette, 1958; Y. Pélicier, 'Aperçus Généraux sur la Psychologie des Transplantés', *Concours Médical*, lxxxvi (1964). See also A. and H. Torrubia, 'Contribution à Une Psychopathologie Sociale, Recherche sur la Transplantation' (for internal migration), *Inst. Nat. d'Hygiène*, Monographie No. 7, Paris, 1955.
10 Cf. SIVADON, 'Géographie Humaine et Psychiatrie', *Annales Médico-Psychologiques*, 106th year (1948).
11 G. DAUMEZON, Y. CHAMPION and J. CHAMPION-BASSET, 'L'Assistance Psychiatrique aux Malades Mentaux d'Origine Nord-africaine Musulmane en France', *Inst. Nat. d'Hygiène*, Monographie No. 14, 1957.
12 Y. PÉLICIER, 'Aperçus Généraux sur la Psychologie des Transplantés', *Concours Médical*, lxxxvi (1964).
13 P. KOECHLIN, 'Perturbations de Méchanismes Instrumentaux d'Insertion au Milieu', *Evol. Psychiat.*, iii (1956).
14 H. DUCHÊNE, 'La Société Vécue', *Evol. Psychiat.*, i (1956).
15 M. K. OPLER, *Culture, Psychiatry and Human Values*, Springfield, Ill., 1956.

16 V. D. SANUA, *op. cit.*

17 M. K. OPLER and B. H. SINGER, 'Ethnic Differences in Behavior and Psychopathology in the Italian and the Irish', *Int. J. Soc. Psychiat.*, ii (1956), pp. 11–12.

18 P. KOECHLIN, *op. cit.*

19 V. V. STANCIU, 'Quelques Suggestions pour Une Hygiène Mentale chez les Immigrés', *Congrès de la Santé Mentale*, Paris, September 1961.

20 G. BOITELLE and C. BOITELLE-LENTULO, *op. cit.*

21 Another phenomenon which has interested French psychiatrists is the greater frequency of *folie à deux* and multiple psychosis among foreigners than among French people, which can be explained by the isolated life of migrant families. See, for example, Bonnafé, Bollette, Gest, Heyward and Sifflet, 'Trois Cas de Délire de Conjoints chez les Transplantés', *XIᵉ Congrès Médec. et Neur. de Langue Française*, Masson, 1953.

22 P. BARRABEE and OTTO VON MERING, 'Ethnic Variation in Mental Stress in Families with Psychotic Children', in Rose, *Mental Health and Mental Disorder: a Sociological Approach*, New York, 1955.

23 HELEN E. FRAZEE, 'Children Who Later Become Schizophrenic', *Smith Coll. Stud. in Soc. Work*, xxiii (1953).

24 R. P. SPERLING, 'A Study of the Psychotic within Three Ethnic Groups', thesis, Harvard, 1953.

25 V. D. SANUA, *op. cit.*

26 RUESCH, JACOBSEN and LOEBE, 'Acculturation and Illness', *Psychol. Monogr.*, lxii, 5 (1948); CHOMBART DE LAUWE, 'La Maladie Mentale comme Phénomène Social', *Monogr. 7 Inst. Nat. d'Hygiène*, 1955.

27 L. LE GUILLANT, 'Psychopathologie de la Transplantation', in A. and H. Torrubia, *op. cit.*

28 SIVADON, *op. cit.*

29 Ombredane gives an example of a remarkable case in Brazil, where the delusion of interpretation arises from misunderstood words. *Etude de Psychologie Médicale*, Vol. III, Rio de Janeiro, 1944, pp. 117–65.

30 Y. PÉLICIER, *op. cit.*, p. 211.

31 A. J. PRANGE, 'An Interpretation of Cultural Isolation and Alien's Paranoid Reaction', *Int. J. Soc. Psychiat.*, iv, 4 (1959).

32 A. KARDINER and L. OUSSAY, *The Mark of Oppression*, New York, 1951.

33 Cf., for example, W. F. WHYTE, *Street Corner Society, the Social Organization of an Italian Slum*, Chicago, 1958.

34 G. BOITELLE and C. BOITELLE-LENTULO, *op. cit.*

35 See Barclay Murphy's chapter in J. McV. Hunt, *Personality and the Behavior Disorders*, New York, 1944.

36 MCBEE, 'A Mental Hygiene Clinic in a High School', *Ment. Hyg.*, xix.

37 Quoted by Y. PÉLICIER, *op. cit.*, p. 163.

38 B. MALZBERG, *op. cit.*, ch. 8.

39 L. E. HINKLE, JR., and H. G. WOLFF, 'Health and the Social Environment, Experimental Investigations', in A. H. Leighton, J. A. Clausen and R. A. Wilson, eds., *Explorations in Social Psychiatry*, New York, 1957.

Chapter VIII The psychiatry of social groups: III. The family

1 JAMES S. BOSSARD, *Social Change and Social Problems*, New York, 2nd Ed., 1938.

2 KATHARINE BEMENT DAVIS, *Factors in the Sex Life of 2,200 Women*, New York, 1929.

3 BENJAMIN MALZBERG, *Social and Biological Aspects of Mental Disease*, New York, 1940, chs. 3 and 4.

4 Literature offers excellent examples of the neurotic's reluctance to marry, e.g. Kierkegaard or Kafka. Schizophrenia is more frequent among bachelors than any other form of mental disorder, according to Malzberg's statistics. The fact that it develops early (hence its old name, dementia praecox) suggests that it is a cause rather than a result of the unmarried state.

5 C. W. WAHL, 'Some Antecedent Factors in the Family Histories of 392 Schizophrenics', *Amer. J. Psychiat.*, cx (1954).

6 V. D. SANUA, *A Comparative Study of Schizophrenics of Different Backgrounds (Italian, Irish, Jews and Protestants)*, Yeshiva University, New York, s.d., mimeograph.

7 ANNEMARIE DUHRSEN, 'Psychiatrische Aspekte zur Familienssoziologie', *Kölner Zeitsch. für Soziol. und Sozialpsych.*, Köln, iii (1958):

	Clinical group	Control group
Mother's family complete	27	34
Mother's family incomplete	23	15
Father's family complete	39	33
Father's family incomplete	11	17

8 DRACONDES, 'Le Développement du Psychisme des Enfants et le Milieu Familial', *Psyché*, v, 45–6 (1950), pp. 580–95.

9 DUHRSEN, *op. cit.*

10 Cf. the special issue of *Revista de Psicologia Normal e Patologica*, São Paulo, Brazil, vi, 4 (1960), devoted to mentally defective children.

11 For a study of these dimensions and others, such as age at the time of bereavement, social class, ethnic group, religion, family size, state of health of the person who dies (whether it is an invalid for whom death is a release from suffering, or a person in the prime of life), see E. H. Volkart, with the collaboration of S. T. Michel, 'Bereavement and Mental Health', in A. H. Leighton, J. A. Clausen and R. N. Wilson, *Explorations in Social Psychiatry*, New York, 1957.

12 J. STROETZEL, *Psychologie Sociale*, Flammarion, 1963.

13 THOMAS D. ELIOT, 'The Bereaved Family', *Ann. Amer. Acad. Pol. and Soc. Sci.*, Philadelphia, 2,501 (1932).

14 S. S. BELLIN and R. H. HARDT, 'Marital Status and Mental Disorders among the Aged', *Amer. Sociol. Rev.*, xxiii, 2 (1958), pp. 155–62.

15 C. W. WAHL, *op. cit.*

16 C. SCHOOLER, 'Birth Order and Schizophrenia', *Arch, Genet. Psychiat.*, iv (1961), pp. 91–4.

17 V. D. SANUA, *op. cit.*

18 B. MALZBERG, *op. cit.*, ch. 10.

19 Alexander also points to disorders in the first-born son in the case of second-generation immigrants, where the mother sacrifices herself to give the child a chance in life, and the father is overshadowed owing to the difficulties of the first generation's achieving success. 'Educative Influences of Personality Factors in the Environment', in C. Kluckhohn and H. A. Murray, *Personality in Nature, Society and Culture*, New York, 1948.

20 GEORGES MAUCO and PAULE RAMBAUD, 'Le Rang de l'Enfant dans la Famille', *Rev. Fr. de Psychanal.*, ii (1951).

21 Cf. DUBLINEAU and FOLLIN, 'Le Bourreau Domestique et le Couple Conjugal; Bases Cliniques d'une Méthodologie Gestaltiste en Charactérologie', *Ann. Méd. Psych.*, i (1944).

22 Cf. ERICK H. ERIKSON, *Childhood and Society*, New York, 1950. For general theory, and for pathological repercussions of child-rearing methods, see Kardiner and Linton, *The Individual and His Society*, New York, 1936.

23 Cf., for example, A. DAVIS and R. J. HAVIGHURST, 'Social Class and Color Differences in Child-rearing', in Kluckhohn and Murray, *op. cit.*

24 E. FROMM, 'Individual and Social Origins of Neurosis', in Kluckhohn and Murray, *op. cit.*

25 RUTH BENEDICT, 'Continuities and Discontinuities in Cultural Conditioning', in Kluckhohn and Murray, *op. cit.*

26 R. J. HAVIGHURST and A. DAVIS, 'A Comparison of the Chicago and Harvard Studies of Social-Class Differences in Child-rearing', *Amer. Sociol. Rev.*, xx, 44 (1955), pp. 438–42.

27 N. CAMERON, 'Role Concepts in Behavior Pathology', *Amer. J. Sociol.*, lv (1950), pp. 464–7.

28 G. BATESON, D. D. JACKSON, J. HALEY and J. WEAKLAND, 'Toward a Theory of Schizophrenia', *Behav. Sci.*, i (1956), pp. 251–64.

29 FRIEDA FROMM-RESCHMANN, 'Notes on the Development of Treatment of Schizophrenia by Psychoanalytic Psychotherapy', *Psychiatry*, xi (1948), pp. 263–73.

30 M. L. KOHN and J. A. CLAUSEN, 'Parental Authority Behavior and Schizophrenia', *Amer. J. Orthopsychiat.*, xxvi (1956), pp. 297–313.

31 HELEN E. FRAZEE, 'Children Who Later Become Schizophrenic', *Smith Coll. Stud. in Soc. Work*, xxiii (1953).

32 P. SIVADON, R. MISES and J. MISES, 'Le Milieu Familial du Schizophrène', *Evol. Psychiat.*, i (1954), pp. 145–57.

33 T. LIDZ, 'The Role of the Father in the Family Environment of the Schizophrenic Patient', *Amer. J. Psychiat.*, cxiii (1951), pp. 126–32.

34 S. ARIETI, *Interpretation of Schizophrenia*, New York, 1955 (summarized by Sanua, *op cit.*).

35 H. M. HITSON and D. H. FUNKESTEIN, 'Family Pattern and Paranoidal Personality in Boston and Burma', *Int. J. Soc. Psychiat.*, v, 3 (1960).

36 V. D. SANUA, *op. cit.*, pp. 37–44.

37 D. L. GÉRARD and J. SIEGEL, 'The Family Background of Schizophrenia', *Psychiat. Quart.*, 1950.

38 LINDESMITH and STRAUSS, 'Critique of Culture-personality Writings', *Amer. Sociol. Rev.*, xv (1950).

39 W. H. SEWELL, 'Infant Training and Personality of the Child', in A. M. Rose, ed., *Mental Health and Mental Disorder, a Sociological Approach*, New York, 1955.

Chapter IX The ordering of the material

1 For example, H. B. MURPHY *et al.*, ed., *Flight and Resettlement*, U.N.E.S.C.O., 1955, showed clearly that mental disturbance in refugees and displaced persons has its roots in the past and not in the vicissitudes of the present. However, these disturbances only break out if the new community does not accept the refugees or remains indifferent to them.

2 RUTH BENEDICT, 'Continuities and Discontinuities in Cultural Conditioning', in Kluckhohn and Murray, *Personality in Nature, Society and Culture*, New York, 1948.

3 PIERRE JANET, 'La Tension psychologique et ses Oscillations', in Dumas, *Traité de Psychologie*, 2 vols., pp. 933–4.

4 CARL R. ROGERS, 'Some Observations on the Organization of Personality', *Amer. Psychol.*, ii (1947), pp. 358–64.

5 DIETHELM, 'The Psychopathologic Basis of Psychotherapy of Schizophrenia', *Symp. Amer. J. Psychiat.*, 1954.

6 Cf. E. MINKOWSKI, *La Schizophrénie, Psychopathologie des Schizoïdes et des Schizophrènes*, Desclée de Brouwer, new ed., 1953.

7 GUNNAR MYRDAL, *An American Dilemma*, Vol. II, Appendix 3: 'A Methodological Note on the Principles of Cumulation', pp. 1065–70, New York, 1944.

8 We would need to quote all his work from the memorandum in *L'Année Sociologique* (on the elementary forms of sociability) onwards. Cf., in particular, *Déterminismes Sociaux et Liberté Humaine*, Presses Universitaires, 1955, and *Dialectique et Sociologie*, Flammarion, 1962.

9 In fact, drug-therapy does not always succeed: 60 per cent of the cases improve, but this still means a 40 per cent failure rate.

10 We must point out here that the importance of 'mothering' (displaying feelings of a maternal nature towards the patient) has been recognized in fields other than pharmacology, by P. C. Recamier, 'Etude Clinique des Frustrations Affectives Précoces', *Rev. Fr. de Psychanal.*, by Courchet in his sociotherapy, by Le Guillant in connection with nurses, etc. But we intend to confine ourselves to the field furthest removed from our own thinking, i.e. psychopharmacology.

11 American literature reports similar findings: cf. G. J. Sarver-Toner, 'Transference and No Specific Drug Effects in the Use of Tranquillizing Drugs', *Amer. Psychiat. Assoc. Res. Report* No. 8 (December 1957).

12 MARCEL MAUSS, 'Rapports Réels et Pratiques de la Psychologie et de la Sociologie', *Journ. de Psychol. Normale et Pathologique*, 1924, and *Sociologie et Anthropologie*, Presses Universitaires, 1950, pp. 294–5, 299–300.

13 CLAUDE LÉVI-STRAUSS, *A World on the Wane*, Eng. tr., 1961.

14 This variability, incidentally, is a justification for all the statistical studies we quoted earlier.

15 LÉVI-STRAUSS, 'Introduction à l'Œuvre de Mauss', in M. Mauss, *Sociologie et Anthropologie, op. cit.*, pp. xx–xxi.

16 S. F. NADEL, 'Shamanism in the Nuba Mountains', *J. Royal Anthrop. Inst.*, lxxvi, Part I (1946).

Chapter X Society and the 'insane'

1 There is an abundant literature on the history of madness. To mention only a few authors, cf. J. Fillozat, *Magie et Civilisation*, P.U.F., 1943; M. Foucault, *Madness and Civilization*, Engl. tr., Tavistock Publications, 1965; Y. Pélicier, *Intégration des Données Sociologiques à la Psychiatrie Clinique*, Masson et Cie., 1964; P. Vallery Radot, *Deux Siècles d'Histoire Hospitalière*, Dupont, 1947.

2 H. EY, *Etudes Psychiatriques*, Desclée de Brouwer, 1948. For a summary of his ideas, see 'Anthropologie du Malade Mental', *Esprit*, xx, 12 (1952).

3 See, for example, BENJAMIN D. PAUL, ed., *Health, Culture and Community*, New York, 1955, J. C. NUNNALLY, JR., *Popular Conceptions of Mental Health, their Development and Change*, New York, 1961, and

numerous other articles, such as J. L. WOODWARD, 'Changing Ideas on Mental Illness and Its Treatment', *Amer. Soc. Rev.*, xvi, 4 (1951), pp. 443–54.

4 Flammarion, 1961. Cf., by the same author, 'Quelques Aspects de la Relation "Malade-médecin" Observés au Cours de Deux Examens Successifs de la Même Malade en Clinique Psychiatrique', *Evol. Psychiat.*, vi, 5 (1953).

5 *Evol. Psychiat.*, ii (1953).

6 JANE PHILIPS, 'Psychodynamique de la Santé et de la Guérison dans les Civilisations, *VIᵉ Congrès Int. des Sc. Anthrop., Ethno.*, II, Vol. 2, Musée de l'Homme (1964), pp. 549–57.

7 'Sur la Parole et le Langage', *La Psychanalyse*, No. 1 (1956).

8 S. H. FOULKES and E. J. ANTHONY, *Group Psychotherapy*, Penguin Books, 1957.

9 J. L. MORENO, *Psychodrama*, I, New York, 1946.

10 P. BALVET, 'Réflexions Dépareillées sur la Psychothérapie', *La Raison*, 1961.

11 M. S. SCHWARZ, 'Social Research in the Mental Hospital', in A. M. Rose, *Mental Health and Mental Disorder: a Sociological Approach*, New York, 1955. On the social life of hospital patients, cf. W. Caudill, in Kroeber, *Anthropology Today*, Chicago, 1953; Caudill, Redlich, H. R. Gilmore and E. B. Brody, 'Social Structure and Interaction Processes on a Psychiatric Ward', *Amer. J. Orthopsychiat.*, xxii (1952); G. Devereux, 'The Social Structure of the Hospital as a Factor in Total Therapy', *ibid.*, xix (1949); H. Warren, Dunham and S. Kirson Weinberg, *The Culture of the State Mental Hospital*, Detroit, 1960; Erving Goffman, *Asylums*, New York, 1961; R. W. Hyde and R. H. York, 'A Technique for Investigating Interpersonal Relationship in a Mental Hospital', *J. Abnorm. Soc. Psychol.*, xliii (1948); Jenkins and Curran, 'The Evolution and Persistence of Groups in a Psychiatric Observation Ward', *J. Soc. Psychol.*, xii (1940); Osorio Cesar, 'Aspectos da Vida Social entre os Loucos', *Rev. Arqu. Munic. de São Paulo*, cv (1946); H. Rowland, 'Interaction Processes in a State Mental Hospital', *Psychiatry*, 1938, and 'Friendship Pattern in a State Mental Hospital', *ibid.*, 1939; Schwartz, 'The Functions of Sociology in the Mental Hospital', *Social Problems*, 1960; Scheimo, Payntor and Szurek, 'Problems of Staff Interaction with Spontaneous Group Formation on a Children's Psychiatric Ward', *Amer. J. Orthopsychiat.*, xix (1949). Stanton and Schwartz, *The Mental Hospital*, New York, 1954, and A. T. Wilson, *Hospital Nursing Auxiliaries, Notes on a Background Survey and Job Analysis*, London, 1951. In France also, in addition to the special issue of *Esprit* 'Misère de la Psychiatrie', xx, 12 (1952), and Courchet's unpublished articles, there are important writings, such as Delay, Maisonneuve, Benda, etc., 'Recherches Psychosociologiques dans un Service Libre de Malades Mentaux', *Ann. Méd. Psych.*, March 1958, or P. C. Récamier, 'Introduction à Une Sociopathie des Schizophrènes Hospitalisés', *Evol. Psychiat.*, i (1957).

12 In particular, Schwartz detected a feed-back circuit between the patient's confusion and disagreement between staff members over his handling. This idea is more closely related to our structuralist approach, since it sees the hospital as a 'split social field'.

13 J. A. DAVIS, H. E. FREEMAN and O. G. SIMMONS, 'Rehospitalization and Performance Level of Former Mental Patients', *Social Problems*, v (1957), pp. 37–44.

14 PARSONS and SHILS, *Toward a General Theory of Action*, Harvard Univ. Press, 1951.
15 H. E. FREEMAN and O. G. SIMMONS, 'Mental Patients in the Community: Family Settings and Performance Levels', *Amer. Sociol. Rev.*, xxiii, 2 (1958), pp. 147–54.
16 T. PARSONS, *Eléments pour Une Sociologie de l'Action*. (This is a collec-tion of readings from Parsons's work, published in French, Chapter 5 of *Eléments* is Chapter 10 of *The Social System*, Routledge & Kegan Paul, 1964.)
17 Ecological studies show that there are undoubtedly zones of deteriora-tion with high concentrations of social problems, but within these zones the delinquency areas are distinct from the areas of mental disorder.
18 To be able to function adequately, a social system has to rely on affec-tive neutrality.

Chapter XI   The world of 'madness'

1 RUESCH and BATESON, *Communication, Social Matrix of Psychiatry*, New York, 1951, and even closer to Blondel, half a century after him, John Cumming and Elaine Cumming, 'Affective Symbolism, Social Norms and Mental Illness', *Psychiatry*, I, 1956.
2 CHARLES MORRIS, *Signs, Language and Behavior*, New York, 1946.
3 P. C. RÉCAMIER, 'Introduction à Une Sociopathologie des Schizophrènes Hospitalisés', *Evol. Psychiat.*, i (1957).
4 KRETSCHMER, *Körperbau und Character*, Berlin, 1940.
5 E. MINKOWSKI, *La Schizophrénie*, Desclée de Brouwer, 1953.
6 E.g. S. K. WEINBERG, 'A Sociological Analysis of a Schizophrenic Type', in Rose, *Mental Health and Mental Disorder: a Sociological Approach*, New York, 1955; G. DEVEREUX, 'A Sociological Theory of Schizophrenia', *Psychoanal. Rev.*, xxvi (1939).
7 NORMAN CAMERON, *The Psychology of Behavior Disorders; a Biosocial Interpretation*, Boston, 1947; 'The Paranoid Pseudo-community', in Rose, *op. cit.*
8 Cf. PIERRE JANET, *De l'Angoisse à l'Extase*, Alcan, 2 vols., 1926 and 1928 (for 'Prince Charming' figures), and O. RANK, 'Der Mythus von der Geburt des Helden', *Schr. zur Angemt. Seelen Kunde*, v, Vienna and Leipzig (1909) (for regal or divine father figures).
9 SEBAG, *Marxisme et Structuralisme*, Paris, Payot, 1964, p. 141.
10 RESNIK, personal communication. J. BOBON and P. ROUMEGUÈRE, 'Du Geste et du Dessin Magiques au Néographisme Conjuratoire', *Acta Neurol. Psychiat. Belgica*, x (1957), pp. 815–29.
11 RALPH LINTON, *The Study of Man*, New York, 1936.
12 G. DEVEREUX, 'Normal and Abnormal', in *Some Uses of Anthropology*, Washington, 1956.
13 *Ibid.*, 'Primitive Psychiatric Diagnosis: a General Theory of the Diag-nostic Process', in *Man's Image in Medicine and Anthropology*.
14 T. J. SCHAFF, 'The Role of the Mentally Ill and the Dynamics of Mental Disorder: a Research Framework', *Sociometry*, iv (1963), pp. 436–53.
15 The finest example of this in psychiatric literature is undoubtedly found in M. A. SECHEHAYE, *La Réalisation Symbolique*, Berne, 1947 (supple-ment of the *Revue Suisse de Psychologie et de Psychologie Appliquée*).
16 FREUD, *Introduction to Psychoanalysis*.
17 From the special issue of *Esprit*, 'Misère de la Psychiatrie', xx, 12 (1952), p. 829.

18 MARCEL MAUSS, 'Effet Physique chez l'Individu de l'Idée de Mort Suggerée par la Collectivité', *Psychol. Norm. Pathol.*, 1926. Also in Mauss, *Sociologie et Anthropologie*, Paris, 1950, pp. 313–30.

19 W. S. INMAN, 'Clinical Observations on Morbid Periodicity', *Brit. J. Med. Psychol.*, xxi, Part 4 (1948), pp. 254–62.

20 E. H. KNIGHT, 'Some Considerations regarding the Concept *"Autism"*', *Dis. Nerv. Syst.*, iv (1965), pp. 224–9.

21 J. BOBON and P. ROUMEGUÈRE, *op. cit.*

22 On the morbid structuring of space, see Minkowski, *op. cit.*, Gabel, *La Réification*, Ed. de Minuit, 1962; A. Arthus, *Le Village*, P. Hartmann, 1949; J. Binswanger, *Le Rêve et l'Existence*, Desclée de Brouwer, 1954; G. Bachelard, *La Poétique de l'Espace*, P.U.F., 1957, etc.

23 DR LAGACHE, personal communication.

24 FREUD, *Metapsychology*.

25 M. KLEIN, *The Psychoanalysis of Children*, London, 1932.

26 A. HESNARD, *Psychanalyse du Lien Interhumain*, P.U.F., 1957, pp. 210–11.

27 A. LAGACHE, 'Contribution à la Psychologie de la Conduite Criminelle', *Rev. Fr. de Psychanal.*, iv (1949), pp. 541–70.

28 H. MICHAUX, *Misérable Miracle*, p. 23.

29 P. B. SCHNEIDER, 'Les Thérapies Psychanalytiques de Groupe', *Rev. Fr. Psychanal.*, xxviii, 6 (1963).

30 H. MENG, 'Psychoses d'Organe', *Psyché*, lvi (1951), pp. 335–49.

31 The first results have appeared in *Neuropsychologie*, i (1963), pp. 165–177.

32 *Totemism*, Engl. tr., ch. 5 (including Durkheim and Mauss's quotation).

33 P. J. BURSZTYN, *Schizophrénie et Mentalité Primitive*, Jouve, 1935.

34 Cf. on this point (but only in relation to the reintegration of 'stabilized' patients into society) G. M. Carstairs, 'The Social Limits of Eccentricity; an English Study', in M. K. Opler, *Culture and Mental Health*, New York, 1959, pp. 373–89.

35 M. HANNER, 'Influence of Small Networks as Factors in Mental Hospital Admission', *Human Organiz.*, xxii, 4 (1963–4), pp. 243–51.

Index

243

247

The International Library of
Sociology
and Social Reconstruction

Edited by W. J. H. SPROTT
Founded by KARL MANNHEIM

ROUTLEDGE & KEGAN PAUL
BROADWAY HOUSE, CARTER LANE, LONDON, E.C.4

CONTENTS

PRINTED IN GREAT BRITAIN BY HEADLEY BROTHERS LTD
109 KINGSWAY LONDON W C 2 AND ASHFORD KENT

GENERAL SOCIOLOGY

Brown, Robert. Explanation in Social Science. *208 pp. 1963. (2nd Impression 1964.) 25s.*

Gibson, Quentin. The Logic of Social Enquiry. *240 pp. 1960. (2nd Impression 1963.) 24s.*

Homans, George C. Sentiments and Activities: Essays in Social Science. *336 pp. 1962. 32s.*

Isajiw, Wsevelod W. Causation and Functionalism in Sociology. *About 192 pp. 1968. 25s.*

Johnson, Harry M. Sociology: a Systematic Introduction. *Foreword by Robert K. Merton. 710 pp. 1961. (4th Impression 1964.) 42s.*

Mannheim, Karl. Essays on Sociology and Social Psychology. *Edited by Paul Keckskemeti. With Editorial Note by Adolph Lowe. 344 pp. 1953. (2nd Impression 1966.) 32s.*

Systematic Sociology: An Introduction to the Study of Society. *Edited by J. S. Erös and Professor W. A. C. Stewart. 220 pp. 1957. (3rd Impression 1967.) 24s.*

Martindale, Don. The Nature and Types of Sociological Theory. *292 pp. 1961. (3rd Impression 1967.) 35s.*

Maus, Heinz. A Short History of Sociology. *234 pp. 1962. (2nd Impression 1965.) 28s.*

Myrdal, Gunnar. Value in Social Theory: A Collection of Essays on Methodology. *Edited by Paul Streeten. 332 pp. 1958. (2nd Impression 1962.) 32s.*

Ogburn, William F., and **Nimkoff, Meyer F.** A Handbook of Sociology. *Preface by Karl Mannheim. 656 pp. 46 figures. 35 tables. 5th edition (revised) 1964. 40s.*

Parsons, Talcott, and **Smelser, Neil J.** Economy and Society: A Study in the Integration of Economic and Social Theory. *362 pp. 1956. (4th Impression 1967.) 35s.*

Rex, John. Key Problems of Sociological Theory. *220 pp. 1961. (4th Impression 1968.) 25s.*

Stark, Werner. The Fundamental Forms of Social Thought. *280 pp. 1962. 32s.*

FOREIGN CLASSICS OF SOCIOLOGY

Durkheim, Emile. Suicide. A Study in Sociology. *Edited and with an Introduction by George Simpson. 404 pp. 1952. (4th Impression 1968.) 35s.*

Socialism and Saint-Simon. *Edited with an Introduction by Alvin W. Gouldner. Translated by Charlotte Sattler from the edition originally edited with an Introduction by Marcel Mauss. 286 pp. 1959. 28s.*

Professional Ethics and Civic Morals. *Translated by Cornelia Brookfield. 288 pp. 1957. 30s.*

Gerth, H. H., and **Mills, C. Wright.** From Max Weber: Essays in Sociology. *502 pp. 1948. (6th Impression 1967.) 35s.*

Tönnies, Ferdinand. Community and Association. *(Gemeinschaft und Gesellschaft.) Translated and Supplemented by Charles P. Loomis. Foreword by Pitirim A. Sorokin. 334 pp. 1955. 28s.*

SOCIAL STRUCTURE

Andreski, Stanislaw. Military Organization and Society. *Foreword by Professor A. R. Radcliffe-Brown. 226 pp. 1 folder. 1954. Revised Edition 1968. 35s.*

Cole, G. D. H. Studies in Class Structure. *220 pp. 1955. (3rd Impression 1964.) 21s.*

Coontz, Sydney H. Population Theories and the Economic Interpretation. *202 pp. 1957. (2nd Impression 1961.) 25s.*

Coser, Lewis. The Functions of Social Conflict. *204 pp. 1956. (3rd Impression 1968.) 25s.*

Dickie-Clark, H. F. Marginal Situation: A Sociological Study of a Coloured Group. *240 pp. 11 tables. 1966. 40s.*

Glass, D. V. (Ed.). Social Mobility in Britain. *Contributions by J. Berent, T. Bottomore, R. C. Chambers, J. Floud, D. V. Glass, J. R. Hall, H. T. Himmelweit, R. K. Kelsall, F. M. Martin, C. A. Moser, R. Mukherjee, and W. Ziegel. 420 pp. 1954. (4th Impression 1967.) 45s.*

Kelsall, R. K. Higher Civil Servants in Britain: From 1870 to the Present Day. *268 pp. 31 tables. 1955. (2nd Impression 1966.) 25s.*

König, René. The Community. *224 pp. 1968. 25s.*

Lawton, Dennis. Social Class, Language and Education. *192 pp. 1968. 21s.*

Marsh, David C. The Changing Social Structure in England and Wales, 1871-1961. *1958. 272 pp. 2nd edition (revised) 1966. (2nd Impression 1967.) 35s.*

Mouzelis, Nicos. Organization and Bureaucracy. An Analysis of Modern Theories. *240 pp. 1967. 28s.*

Ossowski, Stanislaw. Class Structure in the Social Consciousness. *210 pp. 1963. (2nd Impression 1967.) 25s.*

SOCIOLOGY AND POLITICS

Barbu, Zevedei. Democracy and Dictatorship: Their Psychology and Patterns of Life. *300 pp. 1956. 28s.*

Crick, Bernard. The American Science of Politics: Its Origins and Conditions. *284 pp. 1959. 32s.*

Hertz, Frederick. Nationality in History and Politics: A Psychology and Sociology of National Sentiment and Nationalism. *432 pp. 1944. (5th Impression 1966.) 42s.*

Kornhauser, William. The Politics of Mass Society. *272 pp. 20 tables. 1960. (2nd Impression 1965.) 28s.*

Laidler, Harry W. History of Socialism. Social-Economic Movements: An Historical and Comparative Survey of Socialism, Communism, Co-operation, Utopianism; and other Systems of Reform and Reconstruction. *New edition in preparation.*

Lasswell, Harold D. Analysis of Political Behaviour. An Empirical Approach. *324 pp. 1947. (4th Impression 1966.) 35s.*

Mannheim, Karl. Freedom, Power and Democratic Planning. *Edited by Hans Gerth and Ernest K. Bramstedt. 424 pp. 1951. (2nd Impression 1965.) 35s.*

Mansur, Fatma. Process of Independence. *Foreword by A. H. Hanson. 208 pp. 1962. 25s.*

Martin, David A. Pacificism: an Historical and Sociological Study. *262 pp. 1965. 30s.*

Myrdal, Gunnar. The Political Element in the Development of Economic Theory. *Translated from the German by Paul Streeten. 282 pp. 1953. (4th Impression 1965.) 25s.*

Polanyi, Michael. F.R.S. The Logic of Liberty: Reflections and Rejoinders. *228 pp. 1951. 18s.*

Verney, Douglas V. The Analysis of Political Systems. *264 pp. 1959. (3rd Impression 1966.) 28s.*

Wootton, Graham. The Politics of Influence: British Ex-Servicemen, Cabinet Decisions and Cultural Changes, 1917 to 1957. *316 pp. 1963. 30s.*
Workers, Unions and the State. *188 pp. 1966. (2nd Impression 1967.) 25s.*

FOREIGN AFFAIRS: THEIR SOCIAL, POLITICAL AND ECONOMIC FOUNDATIONS

Baer, Gabriel. Population and Society in the Arab East. *Translated by Hanna Szöke. 288 pp. 10 maps. 1964. 40s.*

Bonné, Alfred. State and Economics in the Middle East: A Society in Transition. *482 pp. 2nd (revised) edition 1955. (2nd Impression 1960.) 40s.*
Studies in Economic Development: with special reference to Conditions in the Under-developed Areas of Western Asia and India. *322 pp. 84 tables. 2nd edition 1960. 32s.*

Mayer, J. P. Political Thought in France from the Revolution to the Fifth Republic. *164 pp. 3rd edition (revised) 1961. 16s.*

Trouton, Ruth. Peasant Renaissance in Yugoslavia 1900-1950: A Study of the Development of Yugoslav Peasant Society as affected by Education. *370 pp. 1 map. 1952. 28s.*

CRIMINOLOGY

Ancel, Marc. Social Defence: A Modern Approach to Criminal Problems. *Foreword by Leon Radzinowicz. 240 pp. 1965. 32s.*

Cloward, Richard A., and **Ohlin, Lloyd E.** Delinquency and Opportunity: A Theory of Delinquent Gangs. *248 pp. 1961. 25s.*

Downes, David M. The Delinquent Solution. A Study in Subcultural Theory. *296 pp. 1966. 42s.*

Dunlop, A. B., and **McCabe, S.** Young Men in Detention Centres. *192 pp. 1965. 28s.*

Friedländer, Kate. The Psycho-Analytical Approach to Juvenile Delinquency: Theory, Case Studies, Treatment. *320 pp. 1947. (6th Impression 1967.) 40s.*

5

Glueck, Sheldon and **Eleanor.** Family Environment and Delinquency. *With the statistical assistance of Rose W. Kneznek. 340 pp. 1962. (2nd Impression 1966.) 40s.*

Mannheim, Hermann. Comparative Criminology: a Text Book. *Two volumes. 442 pp. and 380 pp. 1965. (2nd Impression with corrections 1966.) 42s. a volume.*

Morris, Terence. The Criminal Area: A Study in Social Ecology. *Foreword by Hermann Mannheim. 232 pp. 25 tables. 4 maps. 1957. (2nd Impression 1966.) 28s.*

Morris, Terence and **Pauline,** assisted by **Barbara Barer.** Pentonville: A Sociological Study of an English Prison. *416 pp. 16 plates. 1963. 50s.*

Spencer, John C. Crime and the Services. *Foreword by Hermann Mannheim. 336 pp. 1954. 28s.*

Trasler, Gordon. The Explanation of Criminality. *144 pp. 1962. (2nd Impression 1967.) 20s.*

SOCIAL PSYCHOLOGY

Barbu, Zevedei. Problems of Historical Psychology. *248 pp. 1960. 25s.*

Blackburn, Julian. Psychology and the Social Pattern. *184 pp. 1945. (7th Impression 1964.) 16s.*

Fleming, C. M. Adolescence: Its Social Psychology: With an Introduction to recent findings from the fields of Anthropology, Physiology, Medicine, Psychometrics and Sociometry. *288 pp. 2nd edition (revised) 1963. (3rd Impression 1967.) 25s. Paper 12s. 6d.*
The Social Psychology of Education: An Introduction and Guide to Its Study. *136 pp. 2nd edition (revised) 1959. (4th Impression 1967.) 14s. Paper 7s. 6d.*

Halmos, Paul. Towards a Measure of Man: The Frontiers of Normal Adjustment. *276 pp. 1957. 28s.*

Homans, George C. The Human Group. *Foreword by Bernard DeVoto. Introduction by Robert K. Merton. 526 pp. 1951. (7th Impression 1968.) 35s.*
Social Behaviour: its Elementary Forms. *416 pp. 1961. (2nd Impression 1966.) 32s.*

Klein, Josephine. The Study of Groups. *226 pp. 31 figures. 5 tables. 1956. (5th Impression 1967.) 21s. Paper, 9s. 6d.*

Linton, Ralph. The Cultural Background of Personality. *132 pp. 1947. (7th Impression 1968.) 16s.*

Mayo, Elton. The Social Problems of an Industrial Civilization. With an appendix on the Political Problem. *180 pp. 1949. (5th Impression 1966.) 25s.*

Ottaway, A. K. C. Learning Through Group Experience. *176 pp. 1966. 25s.*

Ridder, J. C. de. The Personality of the Urban African in South Africa. A Thematic Apperception Test Study. *196 pp. 12 plates. 1961. 25s.*

Rose, Arnold M. (Ed.). Human Behaviour and Social Processes: an Interactionist Approach. *Contributions by Arnold M. Rose, Ralph H. Turner, Anselm Strauss, Everett C. Hughes, E. Franklin Frazier, Howard S. Becker, et al. 696 pp. 1962. 70s.*

Smelser, Neil J. Theory of Collective Behaviour. *448 pp. 1962. (2nd Impression 1967.) 45s.*

Stephenson, Geoffrey M. The Development of Conscience. *128 pp. 1966. 25s.*

Young, Kimball. Handbook of Social Psychology. *658 pp. 16 figures. 10 tables. 2nd edition (revised) 1957. (3rd Impression 1963.) 40s.*

SOCIOLOGY OF THE FAMILY

Banks, J. A. Prosperity and Parenthood: A study of Family Planning among The Victorian Middle Classes. *262 pp. 1954. (2nd Impression 1965.) 28s.*

Burton, Lindy. Vulnerable Children. *about 272 pp. 1968. 35s.*

Gavron, Hannah. The Captive Wife: Conflicts of Housebound Mothers. *190 pp. 1966. (2nd Impression 1966.) 25s.*

Klein, Josephine. Samples from English Cultures. *1965. (2nd Impression 1967.)*
  1. Three Preliminary Studies and Aspects of Adult Life in England. *447 pp. 50s.*
  2. Child-Rearing Practices and Index. *247 pp. 35s.*

Klein, Viola. Britain's Married Women Workers. *180 pp. 1965. 28s.*

McWhinnie, Alexina M. Adopted Children. How They Grow Up. *304 pp. 1967. (2nd Impression 1968.) 42s.*

Myrdal, Alva and **Klein, Viola.** Women's Two Roles: Home and Work. *238 pp. 27 tables. 1956. Revised Edition 1967. 30s. Paper 15s.*

Parsons, Talcott and **Bales, Robert F.** Family: Socialization and Interaction Process. *In collaboration with James Olds, Morris Zelditch and Philip E. Slater. 456 pp. 50 figures and tables. 1956. (2nd Impression 1964.) 35s.*

THE SOCIAL SERVICES

Ashdown, Margaret and **Brown, S. Clement.** Social Service and Mental Health: An Essay on Psychiatric Social Workers. *280 pp. 1953. 21s.*

Goetschius, George W. Working with Community Groups. *About 256 pp. 1968. about 35s.*

Goetschius, George W. and **Tash, Joan.** Working with Unattached Youth. *416 pp. 1967. 40s.*

Hall, M. Penelope. The Social Services of Modern England. *416 pp. 6th edition (revised) 1963. (2nd Impression with a new Preface 1966.) 30s.*

Hall, M. P., and **Howes, I. V.** The Church in Social Work. A Study of Moral Welfare Work undertaken by the Church of England. *320 pp. 1965. 35s.*

Heywood, Jean S. Children in Care: the Development of the Service for the Deprived Child. *264 pp. 2nd edition (revised) 1965. (2nd Impression 1966.) 32s.*

An Introduction to Teaching Casework Skills. *190 pp. 1964. 28s.*

Jones, Kathleen. Lunacy, Law and Conscience, 1744-1845: the Social History of the Care of the Insane. *268 pp. 1955. 25s.*

Mental Health and Social Policy, 1845-1959. *264 pp. 1960. (2nd Impression 1967.) 28s.*

Jones, Kathleen and **Sidebotham, Roy.** Mental Hospitals at Work. *220 pp. 1962. 30s.*

Kastell, Jean. Casework in Child Care. *Foreword by M. Brooke Willis. 320 pp. 1962. 35s.*

Nokes, P. L. The Professional Task in Welfare Practice. *152 pp. 1967. 28s.*

Rooff, Madeline. Voluntary Societies and Social Policy. *350 pp. 15 tables. 1957. 35s.*

Shenfield, B. E. Social Policies for Old Age: A Review of Social Provision for Old Age in Great Britain. *260 pp. 39 tables. 1957. 25s.*

Timms, Noel. Psychiatric Social Work in Great Britain (1939-1962). *280 pp. 1964. 32s.*

Social Casework: Principles and Practice. *256 pp. 1964. (2nd Impression 1966.) 25s. Paper 15s.*

Trasler, Gordon. In Place of Parents: A Study in Foster Care. *272 pp. 1960. (2nd Impression 1966.) 30s.*

Young, A. F., and **Ashton, E. T.** British Social Work in the Nineteenth Century. *288 pp. 1956. (2nd Impression 1963.) 28s.*

Young, A. F. Social Services in British Industry. *about 350 pp. 1968. about 45s.*

SOCIOLOGY OF EDUCATION

Banks, Olive. Parity and Prestige in English Secondary Education: a Study in Educational Sociology. *272 pp. 1955. (2nd Impression 1963.) 32s.*

Bentwich, Joseph. Education in Israel. *224 pp. 8 pp. plates. 1965. 24s.*

Blyth, W. A. L. English Primary Education. A Sociological Description. *1965. Revised edition 1967.*
  1. Schools. *232 pp. 30s.*
  2. Background. *168 pp. 25s.*

Collier, K. G. The Social Purposes of Education: Personal and Social Values in Education. *268 pp. 1959. (3rd Impression 1965.) 21s.*

Dale, R. R., and **Griffith, S.** Down Stream: Failure in the Grammar School. *108 pp. 1965. 20s.*

Dore, R. P. Education in Tokugawa Japan. *356 pp. 9 pp. plates. 1965. 35s.*

Edmonds, E. L. The School Inspector. *Foreword by Sir William Alexander. 214 pp. 1962. 28s.*

Evans, K. M. Sociometry and Education. *158 pp. 1962. (2nd Impression 1966.) 18s.*

Foster, P. J. Education and Social Change in Ghana. *336 pp. 3 maps. 1965.* (*2nd Impression 1967.*) *36s.*

Fraser, W. R. Education and Society in Modern France. *150 pp. 1963. 20s.*

Hans, Nicholas. New Trends in Education in the Eighteenth Century. *278 pp. 19 tables. 1951.* (*2nd Impression 1966.*) *30s.*
   Comparative Education: A Study of Educational Factors and Traditions. *360 pp. 3rd (revised) edition 1958.* (*4th Impression 1967.*) *25s. Paper 12s. 6d.*

Hargreaves, David. Social Relations in a Secondary School. *240 pp. 1967. 32s.*

Holmes, Brian. Problems in Education. A Comparative Approach. *336 pp. 1965.* (*2nd Impression 1967.*) *32s.*

Mannheim, Karl and **Stewart, W. A. C.** An Introduction to the Sociology of Education. *206 pp. 1962.* (*2nd Impression 1965.*) *21s.*

Musgrove, F. Youth and the Social Order. *176 pp. 1964. 21s.*

Ortega y Gasset, José. Mission of the University. *Translated with an Introduction by Howard Lee Nostrand. 86 pp. 1946.* (*3rd Impression 1963.*) *15s.*

Ottaway, A. K. C. Education and Society: An Introduction to the Sociology of Education. *With an Introduction by W. O. Lester Smith. 212 pp. Second edition (revised). 1962.* (*5th Impression 1968.*) *18s. Paper 10s. 6d.*

Peers, Robert. Adult Education: A Comparative Study. *398 pp. 2nd edition 1959.* (*2nd Impression 1966.*) *42s.*

Pritchard, D. G. Education and the Handicapped: 1760 to 1960. *258 pp. 1963.* (*2nd Impression 1966.*) *35s.*

Simon, Brian and **Joan** (Eds.). Educational Psychology in the U.S.S.R. *Introduction by Brian and Joan Simon. Translation by Joan Simon. Papers by D. N. Bogoiavlenski and N. A. Menchinskaia, D. B. Elkonin, E. A. Fleshner, Z. I. Kalmykova, G. S. Kostiuk, V. A. Krutetski, A. N. Leontiev, A. R. Luria, E. A. Milerian, R. G. Natadze, B. M. Teplov, L. S. Vygotski, L. V. Zankov. 296 pp. 1963. 40s.*

SOCIOLOGY OF CULTURE

Eppel, E. M., and **M.** Adolescents and Morality: A Study of some Moral Values and Dilemmas of Working Adolescents in the Context of a changing Climate of Opinion. *Foreword by W. J. H. Sprott. 268 pp. 39 tables. 1966. 30s.*

Fromm, Erich. The Fear of Freedom. *286 pp. 1942.* (*8th Impression 1960.*) *25s. Paper 10s.*
   The Sane Society. *400 pp. 1956.* (*3rd Impression 1963.*) *28s. Paper 12s. 6d.*

Mannheim, Karl. Diagnosis of Our Time: Wartime Essays of a Sociologist. *208 pp. 1943.* (*8th Impression 1966.*) *21s.*
   Essays on the Sociology of Culture. *Edited by Ernst Mannheim in co-operation with Paul Kecskemeti. Editorial Note by Adolph Lowe. 280 pp. 1956.* (*3rd Impression 1967.*) *28s.*

Weber, Alfred. Farewell to European History: or The Conquest of Nihilism. *Translated from the German by R. F. C. Hull. 224 pp. 1947. 18s.*

SOCIOLOGY OF RELIGION

Argyle, Michael. Religious Behaviour. *224 pp. 8 figures. 41 tables. 1958. (3rd Impression 1965.) 25s.*

Knight, Frank H., and **Merriam, Thornton W.** The Economic Order and Religion. *242 pp. 1947. 18s.*

Stark, Werner. The Sociology of Religion. A Study of Christendom.
Volume I. Established Religion. *248 pp. 1966. 35s.*
Volume II. Sectarian Religion. *368 pp. 1967. 40s.*
Volume III. The Universal Church. *464 pp. 1967. 45s.*

Watt, W. Montgomery. Islam and the Integration of Society. *320 pp. 1961. (3rd Impression 1966.) 35s.*

SOCIOLOGY OF ART AND LITERATURE

Beljame, Alexandre. Men of Letters and the English Public in the Eighteenth Century: 1660-1744, Dryden, Addison, Pope. *Edited with an Introduction and Notes by Bonamy Dobrée. Translated by E. O. Lorimer. 532 pp. 1948. 32s.*

Misch, Georg. A History of Autobiography in Antiquity. *Translated by E. W. Dickes. 2 Volumes. Vol. 1, 364 pp., Vol. 2, 372 pp. 1950. 45s. the set.*

Schücking, L. L. The Sociology of Literary Taste. *112 pp. 2nd (revised) edition 1966. 18s.*

Silbermann, Alphons. The Sociology of Music. *Translated from the German by Corbet Stewart. 222 pp. 1963. 28s.*

SOCIOLOGY OF KNOWLEDGE

Mannheim, Karl. Essays on the Sociology of Knowledge. *Edited by Paul Kecskemeti. Editorial note by Adolph Lowe. 352 pp. 1952. (3rd Impression 1964.) 35s.*

Stark, W. America: Ideal and Reality. The United States of 1776 in Contemporary Philosophy. *136 pp. 1947. 12s.*
The Sociology of Knowledge: An Essay in Aid of a Deeper Understanding of the History of Ideas. *384 pp. 1958. (3rd Impression 1967.) 36s.*
Montesquieu: Pioneer of the Sociology of Knowledge. *244 pp. 1960. 25s.*

URBAN SOCIOLOGY

Anderson, Nels. The Urban Community: A World Perspective. *532 pp. 1960. 35s.*

Ashworth, William. The Genesis of Modern British Town Planning: A Study in Economic and Social History of the Nineteenth and Twentieth Centuries. *288 pp. 1954. (3rd Impression 1968.) 32s.*

Bracey, Howard. Neighbours: On New Estates and Subdivisions in England and U.S.A. *220 pp. 1964. 28s.*

Cullingworth, J. B. Housing Needs and Planning Policy: A Restatement of the Problems of Housing Need and "Overspill" in England and Wales. *232 pp. 44 tables. 8 maps. 1960. (2nd Impression 1966.) 28s.*

Dickinson, Robert E. City and Region: A Geographical Interpretation. *608 pp. 125 figures. 1964. (5th Impression 1967.) 60s.*

The West European City: A Geographical Interpretation. *600 pp. 129 maps. 29 plates. 2nd edition 1962. (3rd Impression 1968.) 55s.*

The City Region in Western Europe. *320 pp. Maps. 1967. 30s. Paper 14s.*

Jennings, Hilda. Societies in the Making: a Study of Development and Redevelopment within a County Borough. *Foreword by D. A. Clark. 286 pp. 1962. (2nd Impression 1967.) 32s.*

Kerr, Madeline. The People of Ship Street. *240 pp. 1958. 23s.*

Mann, P. H. An Approach to Urban Sociology. *240 pp. 1965. (2nd Impression 1968.) 30s.*

Morris, R. N., and **Mogey, J.** The Sociology of Housing. Studies at Berinsfield. *232 pp. 4 pp. plates. 1965. 42s.*

Rosser, C., and **Harris, C.** The Family and Social Change. A Study of Family and Kinship in a South Wales Town. *352 pp. 8 maps. 1965. (2nd Impression 1968.) 45s.*

RURAL SOCIOLOGY

Haswell, M. R. The Economics of Development in Village India. *120 pp. 1967. 21s.*

Littlejohn, James. Westrigg: the Sociology of a Cheviot Parish. *172 pp. 5 figures. 1963. 25s.*

Williams, W. M. The Country Craftsman: A Study of Some Rural Crafts and the Rural Industries Organization in England. *248 pp. 9 figures. 1958. 25s. (Dartington Hall Studies in Rural Sociology.)*

The Sociology of an English Village: Gosforth. *272 pp. 12 figures. 13 tables. 1956. (3rd Impression 1964.) 25s.*

SOCIOLOGY OF MIGRATION

Eisenstadt, S. N. The Absorption of Immigrants: a Comparative Study based mainly on the Jewish Community in Palestine and the State of Israel. *288 pp. 1954. 28s.*

Humphreys, Alexander J. New Dubliners: Urbanization and the Irish Family. *Foreword by George C. Homans. 304 pp. 1966. 40s.*

SOCIOLOGY OF INDUSTRY AND DISTRIBUTION

Anderson, Nels. Work and Leisure. *280 pp. 1961. 28s.*

Blau, Peter M., and **Scott, W. Richard.** Formal Organizations: a Comparative approach. *Introduction and Additional Bibliography by J. H. Smith. 326 pp. 1963. (2nd Impression 1964.) 28s. Paper 15s.*

Eldridge, J. E. T. Industrial Disputes. Essays in the Sociology of Industrial Relations. *about 272 pp. 1968. 40s.*

Hollowell, Peter G. The Lorry Driver. *272 pp. 1968. 42s.*

Jefferys, Margot, with the assistance of Winifred Moss. Mobility in the Labour Market: Employment Changes in Battersea and Dagenham. *Preface by Barbara Wootton. 186 pp. 51 tables. 1954. 15s.*

Levy, A. B. Private Corporations and Their Control. *Two Volumes. Vol. 1, 464 pp., Vol. 2, 432 pp. 1950. 80s. the set.*

Liepmann, Kate. Apprenticeship: An Enquiry into its Adequacy under Modern Conditions. *Foreword by H. D. Dickinson. 232 pp. 6 tables. 1960. (2nd Impression 1960.) 23s.*

Millerson, Geoffrey. The Qualifying Associations: a Study in Professionalization. *320 pp. 1964. 42s.*

Smelser, Neil J. Social Change in the Industrial Revolution: An Application of Theory to the Lancashire Cotton Industry, 1770-1840. *468 pp. 12 figures. 14 tables. 1959. (2nd Impression 1960.) 42s.*

Williams, Gertrude. Recruitment to Skilled Trades. *240 pp. 1957. 23s.*

Young, A. F. Industrial Injuries Insurance: an Examination of British Policy. *192 pp. 1964. 30s.*

ANTHROPOLOGY

Ammar, Hamed. Growing up in an Egyptian Village: Silwa, Province of Aswan. *336 pp. 1954. (2nd Impression 1966.) 35s.*

Crook, David and **Isabel.** Revolution in a Chinese Village: Ten Mile Inn. *230 pp. 8 plates. 1 map. 1959. 21s.*
The First Years of Yangyi Commune. *302 pp. 12 plates. 1966. 42s.*

Dickie-Clark, H. F. The Marginal Situation. A Sociological Study of a Coloured Group. *236 pp. 1966. 40s.*

Dube, S. C. Indian Village. *Foreword by Morris Edward Opler. 276 pp. 4 plates. 1955. (5th Impression 1965.) 25s.*
India's Changing Villages: Human Factors in Community Development. *260 pp. 8 plates. 1 map. 1958. (3rd Impression 1963.) 25s.*

Firth, Raymond. Malay Fishermen. Their Peasant Economy. *420 pp. 17 pp. plates. 2nd edition revised and enlarged 1966. (2nd Impression 1968.) 55s.*

Gulliver, P. H. The Family Herds. A Study of two Pastoral Tribes in East Africa, The Jie and Turkana. *304 pp. 4 plates. 19 figures. 1955. (2nd Impression with new preface and bibliography 1966.) 35s.*
Social Control in an African Society: a Study of the Arusha, Agricultural Masai of Northern Tanganyika. *320 pp. 8 plates. 10 figures. 1963. 35s.*

Hogbin, Ian. Transformation Scene. The Changing Culture of a New Guinea Village. *340 pp. 22 plates. 2 maps. 1951. 30s.*

Ishwaran, K. Shivapur. A South Indian Village. *about 216 pp. 1968. 35s.*
Tradition and Economy in Village India: An Interactionist Approach. *Foreword by Conrad Arensburg. 176 pp. 1966. 25s.*

Jarvie, Ian C. The Revolution in Anthropology. *268 pp. 1964. (2nd Impression 1967.) 40s.*

Jarvie, Ian C. and **Agassi, Joseph.** Hong Kong. A Society in Transition. *about 388 pp. 1968. 56s.*

Little, Kenneth L. Mende of Sierra Leone. *308 pp. and folder. 1951. Revised edition 1967. 63s.*

Lowie, Professor Robert H. Social Organization. *494 pp. 1950. (4th Impression 1966.) 42s.*

Maunier, René. The Sociology of Colonies: An Introduction to the Study of Race Contact. *Edited and translated by E. O. Lorimer. 2 Volumes. Vol. 1, 430 pp. Vol. 2, 356 pp. 1949. 70s. the set.*

Mayer, Adrian C. Caste and Kinship in Central India: A Village and its Region. *328 pp. 16 plates. 15 figures. 16 tables. 1960. (2nd Impression 1965.) 35s.*
Peasants in the Pacific: A Study of Fiji Indian Rural Society. *232 pp. 16 plates. 10 figures. 14 tables. 1961. 35s.*

Smith, Raymond T. The Negro Family in British Guiana: Family Structure and Social Status in the Villages. *With a Foreword by Meyer Fortes. 314 pp. 8 plates. 1 figure. 4 maps. 1956. (2nd Impression 1965.) 35s.*

DOCUMENTARY

Meek, Dorothea L. (Ed.). Soviet Youth: Some Achievements and Problems. *Excerpts from the Soviet Press, translated by the editor. 280 pp. 1957. 28s.*

Schlesinger, Rudolf (Ed.). Changing Attitudes in Soviet Russia.

1. The Family in the U.S.S.R. *Documents and Readings, with an Introduction by the editor. 434 pp. 1949. 30s.*

2. The Nationalities Problem and Soviet Administration. Selected Readings on the Development of Soviet Nationalities Policies. *Introduced by the editor. Translated by W. W. Gottlieb. 324 pp. 1956. 30s.*

Reports of the Institute of Community Studies

(Demy 8vo.)

Cartwright, Ann. Human Relations and Hospital Care. *272 pp. 1964. 30s.*

Patients and their Doctors. A Study of General Practice. *304 pp. 1967. 40s.*

Jackson, Brian. Streaming: an Education System in Miniature. *168 pp. 1964. (2nd Impression 1966.) 21s. Paper 10s.*

Working Class Community. Some General Notions raised by a Series of Studies in Northern England. *192 pp. 1968. 25s.*

Jackson, Brian and **Marsden, Dennis.** Education and the Working Class: Some General Themes raised by a Study of 88 Working-class Children in a Northern Industrial City. *268 pp. 2 folders. 1962. (4th Impression 1968.) 32s.*

Marris, Peter. Widows and their Families. *Foreword by Dr. John Bowlby. 184 pp. 18 tables. Statistical Summary. 1958. 18s.*

Family and Social Change in an African City. A Study of Rehousing in Lagos. *196 pp. 1 map. 4 plates. 53 tables. 1961. (2nd Impression 1966.) 30s.*

The Experience of Higher Education. *232 pp. 27 tables. 1964. 25s.*

Marris, Peter and **Rein, Martin.** Dilemmas of Social Reform. Poverty and Community Action in the United States. *256 pp. 1967. 35s.*

Mills, Enid. Living with Mental Illness: a Study in East London. *Foreword by Morris Carstairs. 196 pp. 1962. 28s.*

Runciman, W. G. Relative Deprivation and Social Justice. A Study of Attitudes to Social Inequality in Twentieth Century England. *352 pp. 1966. (2nd Impression 1967.) 40s.*

Townsend, Peter. The Family Life of Old People: An Inquiry in East London. *Foreword by J. H. Sheldon. 300 pp. 3 figures. 63 tables. 1957. (3rd Impression 1967.) 30s.*

Willmott, Peter. Adolescent Boys in East London. *230 pp. 1966. 30s.*

The Evolution of a Community: a study of Dagenham after forty years. *168 pp. 2 maps. 1963. 21s.*

Willmott, Peter and **Young, Michael.** Family and Class in a London Suburb. *202 pp. 47 tables. 1960. (4th Impression 1968.) 25s.*

Young, Michael. Innovation and Research in Education. *192 pp. 1965. 25s.*

Young, Michael and **McGeeney, Patrick.** Learning Begins at Home. A Study of a Junior School and its Parents. *about 128 pp. 1968. about 18s. Paper about 8s.*

Young, Michael and **Willmott, Peter.** Family and Kinship in East London. *Foreword by Richard M. Titmuss. 252 pp. 39 tables. 1957. (3rd Impression 1965.) 28s.*

The British Journal of Sociology. *Edited by Terence P. Morris. Vol. 1, No. 1, March 1950 and Quarterly. Roy. 8vo., £2 10s. annually, 15s. a number, post free. (Vols. 1-16, £6 each; Vol. 17, £2 10s. Individual parts 37s. 6d. and 15s. respectively.)*

All prices are net and subject to alteration without notice